THE
MOUTH⇔BODY
CONNECTION

THE MOUTH⇔BODY CONNECTION

A 28-DAY PROGRAM TO CREATE A HEALTHY MOUTH,
REDUCE INFLAMMATION, AND PREVENT DISEASE
THROUGHOUT THE BODY

Gerald P. Curatola D.D.S.
with
Diane Reverand

CENTER
STREET

NEW YORK   NASHVILLE

Copyright © 2017 by Gerald Curatola D.D.S.
Cover design by Julee Brand. Cover Photograph courtesy of Dan Demetriad. Cover copyright © 2017 by Hachette Book Group, Inc.

Center Street
Hachette Book Group
1290 Avenue of the Americas, New York, NY 10104
centerstreet.com
twitter.com/centerstreet

First Hardcover Edition: June 2017

Center Street is a division of Hachette Book Group, Inc. The Center Street name and logo are trademarks of Hachette Book Group, Inc.

The publisher is not responsible for websites (or their content) that are not owned by the publisher.

The Hachette Speakers Bureau provides a wide range of authors for speaking events. To find out more, go to www.HachetteSpeakersBureau.com or call (866) 376-6591.

Illustrations by Josh McKible
Library of Congress Cataloging-in-Publication Data has been applied for.

ISBNs: 978-1-5460-8254-5 (hardcover), 978-1-4789-6971-6 (audiobook, downloadable), 978-1-4789-6970-9 (Audiobook, CD), 978-1-5460-8253-8 (ebook)

Printed in the United States of America

LSC-C

10 9 8 7 6 5 4 3 2 1

To my amazing wife of three decades, Georgia, who has been a "rock solid" soul mate with positive advice, encouragement, and tireless support.

To my three children, Gia, Grant, and Grace, who are my dearest friends and my "advisory team," always giving loving, honest, and caring feedback.

To my mentors, teachers, friends, and colleagues, a "band of brothers and sisters" who have generously shared on the health and wellness paths we travel together.

Most of all, this book is dedicated to God, who gave me the faith to believe in the answer to a childhood prayer, "What should I be when I grow up?"

The answer came and what immediately followed at age six was the dentist's business card I made with scissors, scotch tape, a pen, and one of my father's old business cards.

I am thankful every day for this noble calling, and the many blessings that have followed.

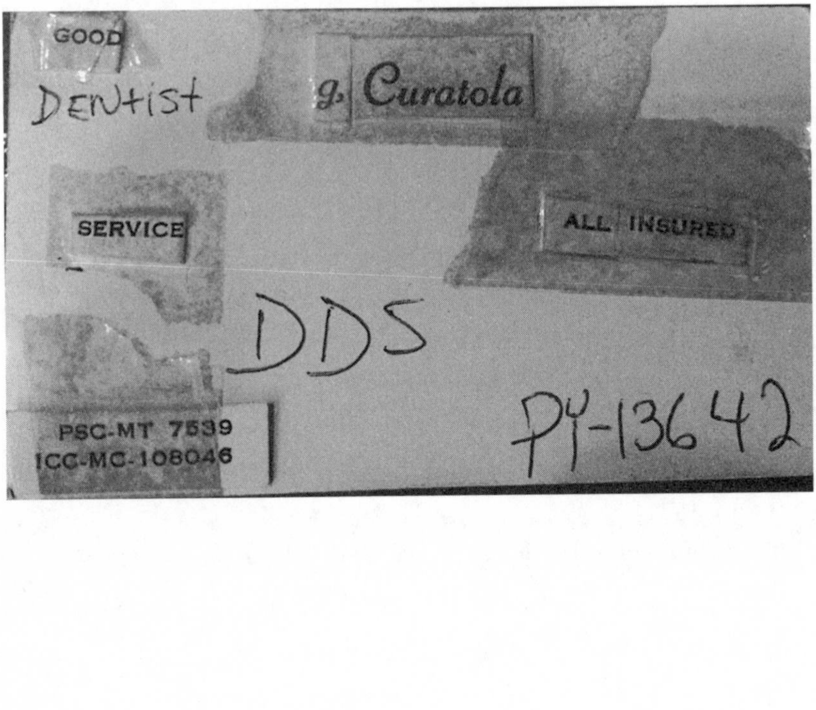
GOOD
DENtist
g. Curatola
SERVICE
ALL INSURED
DDS
PSC-MT 7539
ICC-MC-108046
PY-13642

A Note from the Author

My patients often ask me if I made up my name, which means "cure all." Though I was born with the name, the concept has been the driving force of my career. Working as an oral health expert and wellness pioneer for more than thirty years, my approach at Rejuvenation Dentistry is integrative and restorative.

I have done post-doctoral training in complementary and alternative medicine and integrative nutrition to look at the big picture, the whole body, so that I can give my patients the best care. Everything that happens in the body is interconnected. If something is off in one system, it has to affect others. I like to say that the mouth is both a gateway to the body and a mirror. Your mouth offers direct access to the rest of your body and, at the same time, reflects what is going on inside.

Current research has associated chronic low-grade inflammation in the mouth with a host of chronic illnesses. All too often I have seen gum disease accompany other illnesses such as diabetes and cardiovascular disease. As you will read later, this can be a "which comes first—chicken or egg?" situation. Either way, gum disease is an important marker for problems in the rest of your body.

I become more convinced every day that the principle behind wellness is balance. The complex interplay of all the systems that make your body work requires intricate balance. Disruption in any one system requires adjustments in all of them. Your body automatically seeks equilibrium, which is known as homeostasis. When your equilibrium is disturbed, all your systems are stressed. *The Mouth⇔Body Connection* explores how the condition of your mouth affects your whole body and what you can do to support the balance you need to be healthy.

When a patient comes to me with or without oral disease, I take a full history: chronic illnesses, medications, diet, exercise, stress levels, alcohol consumption, and smoking. Having cared for thousands of people, I have learned that oral health depends on a lot more than hygiene. Nutrition, exercise, and stress reduction all play as big a part in the health of teeth and gums as they do for the entire body. Over the years, I have developed a program to help my patients reverse and prevent gum disease and improve their overall health in the process. I have taken the latest research and converted those findings to practical action.

I decided to write this book for those of you who are not able to see me at my New York City office, so that you will understand and learn to manage the powerful connection between your mouth and your body. I want to share the three-stage Curatola Care Program, which has worked well for my patients. The benefits of my comprehensive program are far-reaching. Research has shown that what works for restoring balance to the mouth also works for the entire body, and what works for the body will improve the balance in the mouth. The 28-Day Curatola Care Program focuses on "getting the junk out of the trunk," by recognizing and eliminating the toxins in your life that are inflaming your gums and your body, following a plan designed to reduce that inflammation and to restore balance, and embracing a way of life that will keep you healthy.

If you resolve to follow the 28-Day Curatola Care Program laid out in *The Mouth⇔Body Connection*, you will be on track to raising your energy, your spirits, and your quality of life, because bringing your body back to its natural balance has a big payoff. You will look and feel your best and be ready to greet each day with a brilliant smile.

Dr. Gerry Curatola
New York, New York
September 2016

Contents

Mouth Matters

Do you know what the following diseases have in common?

- Cardiovascular disease
- Stroke
- Rheumatoid arthritis
- Alzheimer's disease
- Type 2 diabetes
- Obesity
- Metabolic syndrome
- Respiratory tract infections
- Pneumonia
- Asthma
- Hay fever
- COPD
- Premature birth
- Stillbirth
- Colorectal cancer
- Pancreatic cancer
- Lung cancer
- Leukemia
- Kidney cancer
- Mouth, throat, jaw, tongue cancer
- Inflammatory bowel disease

- Osteoporosis
- Erectile dysfunction

You would be right if you realized that inflammation is involved in all of these diseases. Recent research has revealed a more specific connection: Links have been found between each of these illnesses and gum disease. **The health of your mouth appears to have a profound impact on the rest of your body. Even low-grade gum disease has been associated with serious systemic problems.**

Chronic oral disease, which may persist undetected for years, is a major source of low-grade inflammation in the entire body. Inflammation is a defensive biological reaction to a harmful agent. The pain, redness, and swelling that follow a bee sting are signs of acute inflammation. The body is protecting itself to remove irritants, damaged cells, or pathogens, so that the healing process can begin. Chronic inflammation is different. A low-intensity irritant that persists causes long-term inflammation. The irritant can be the sugar and chemicals in processed foods, the stress of your life, a sedentary lifestyle, or working out too hard. When your body is in an inflamed state, it is out of balance. Energy is constantly expended in an attempt to get rid of or adjust to the presence of a perceived irritant. When chronically inflamed, your body is on alert to defend itself. Being in this state for extended periods interferes with the normal function of your body's various systems and wears you down.

According to the *New York Times*, the results of a major survey showed that more than 75 percent of American adults have some form of chronic gum disease, and that only 60 percent of those affected have any knowledge of the problem. That means that **at least 30 percent of the adults in the United States are unaware that their mouths are ticking time bombs that could potentially undermine their health, and another 45 percent might or might not be dealing with their condition.**

During the past ten years, there has been a significant shift in perspective on the connection between oral and systemic health. Research has been shining a light on the impact diseases of the mouth have on the rest of the body. Everything we knew about the causes and origins of disease has been turned upside down by the new field of microbionics, the emerging science of the microbiome, the communities of microorganisms that inhabit your body. *The Mouth⇔Body Connection* focuses on the oral microbiome, which both affects and reflects your overall health.

Part 1 gives you the scientific background for understanding the mouth⇔body connection. You will never look at illness the same way after my crash course on the microbiome. By focusing on oral microbial communities, I establish the bidirectional nature of the mouth, which is both a mirror and a gateway. I move on to cover what can go wrong in your mouth when your microbiome is disturbed. From hijacking the immune system to health-destroying inflammation, I focus on how an unbalanced microbial colony in your mouth can affect oral and overall health. The first part of the book covers up-to-the-minute research on the oral-systemic connection.

I also hit on one of my favorite subjects: the ecological catastrophe in your mouth brought on by antiseptic toothpastes and mouthwashes. The antimicrobial movement in dental care is literally overkill. Using conventional oral care products wipes out your entire oral microbiome, taking the good microbes along with the bad. My position against this scorched earth policy is revolutionary. After all, companies that produce personal care products spend millions of dollars to sell their products with the promise that they "kill germs on contact." That statement is not false advertising. The issue is whether that is a desirable effect.

I argue that there is a connection between sterilizing the mouth, which became popular in the 1970s, and the catastrophic rise we have witnessed in diseases like obesity, diabetes, cardiovascular disease, and metabolic syndrome. Of course, many factors are responsible for the epidemic proportions these illnesses have reached, but rendering the oral microbiome ineffective in its protective role and creating a climate in the mouth in which pathogens thrive certainly contribute to the health crisis today. For the past ten years, I have worked on developing Revitin®, a toothpaste designed to sustain a healthy oral microbiome.

Once you have grasped the importance of the mouth⇔body connection, you will no doubt be ready to do something about it. Part 2 of the book is an overview of how to restore balance in your body. These chapters explain the rationale for the Curatola Care Program and cover the fundamentals for fighting inflammation. As always, before beginning any program or diet, you should run it by your doctor. My program is not like a fad diet that you follow for a set period of time and then go back to "normal." The Curatola Care Program is about making permanent changes in the way you live—how you foster a healthy oral microbiome, what you eat, how you incorporate exercise into your life, and how you deal with stress. The program is designed to help you change habits that are undermining your health and replace them with ways to keep your microbiome in balance. You will feel the difference in just twenty-eight days. My patients do. They sleep better, have more energy, and experience an elevation in mood.

It starts with an oral detox, which includes removing chemicals that have a toxic effect on your teeth and gums. I look at toxic ingredients in toothpaste and mouthwash that are meant to promote oral health. Even "natural" toothpastes have questionable ingredients. I address the controversial issue of fluoride, which has been shown to affect the thyroid, cause weight gain, and lower IQ in children, among other negative effects. I discuss medications that can mess with your oral health and other risk factors. I explain how your fillings can be poisoning your body.

The next step in the plan is nutrition. The Triple A Diet—anti-inflammatory, alkalizing, antioxidant—will create a balanced environment that supports a healthy microbiome. I explain why simple carbohydrates are a disaster for the mouth and how they turn the mouth and body acidic, a state that promotes disease. I also recommend supplements that will help to support the changes you are going to make in your diet and supply the nutrients you need to fight inflammation.

Adding more of the right movement to your life is an important part of the plan. Studies have shown that oral microbiomes of sedentary people are often out of balance. Though exercise can quiet the stress response, too much exercise can cause inflammation. Working out for hours in the gym doing cardio and strength training is not necessary on my plan. In fact, it is not a good idea if you want a healthy mouth. It's all about intensity. Only fifteen minutes of high-intensity resistance training twice a week will do the trick—and it can be done anywhere. There are no excuses—anyone can find thirty minutes a week—two fifteen-minute workouts—to lock in the health benefits of regular exercise. Adam Zickerman, owner of InForm Fitness and author of the *New York Times* bestseller *Power of 10*, has designed simple, high-intensity workouts especially for *The Mouth⇔Body Connection* that can be done anywhere. You also have to build more movement into your life, and Adam gives you simple ways to increase your level of activity.

In order to sustain the balance you achieve, you need some stress management techniques up your sleeve. To do all I want to do, I have had to become expert at stress management. Life's demands keep the pressure on nonstop, and stress has a destructive effect on the entire microbial community in your body. I can tell by examining patients' mouths how stressed out they are. Canker sores are a dead giveaway. Stress can lead to teeth grinding and clenching teeth, which is called bruxism. The pressure of grinding your teeth can wear down the tips of your teeth, flattening them. Habitual grinding rubs off enamel, which makes your teeth more sensitive. Sometimes I observe indentations in the tongues of patients who grind. The same action can affect the joints and muscles in the jaws and neck. I often hear complaints from the super-stressed that involve jaw pain and popping and clicking of the jaw. Stress, which can dry out your mouth, can lead to gum disease as well. The Curatola Care Program offers a variety of relaxation techniques and guidelines for tapping into your body's relaxation response to calm your chronic stress and to reduce the inflammation that chronic stress can cause.

Part 3 puts all the fundamentals together in an easy-to-follow program that leaves out the guesswork. The 28-Day Curatola Care Program gives you a week-by-week guide to preserving or restoring balance in your body. I designed the program to be four weeks long, because twenty-eight days are enough time for a new habit to take root. Though you might not completely lock it in in a month, the program will get you on the road to balance. The Curatola Care Program is not one that you are "on" for twenty-eight days and then go "off." My goal is to encourage you to make some fundamental changes in the way you live for lasting health and well-being, not to mention a brighter smile.

The program is divided into three levels plus bonus emergency remedies and advice:

WEEK 1: RETHINK/CLEAN UP

You start the cleanup program by replacing harsh toothpaste and mouthwash with homemade or recommended alternatives. You will begin to eliminate inflammatory foods, take supplements to counter sugar/simple carbohydrate withdrawal, exercise efficiently, and build some focused relaxation time into each day. A detailed meal plan for the week to help your body detoxify is included as well as a suggested daily schedule.

WEEKS 2 AND 3: RESTORE/SHIFT THE BALANCE

Adding anti-inflammatory foods and those that support a well-balanced microbiome in your mouth and your gut is a big part of this stage. Supplements are suggested to help you make the transition. Meal plans for this two-week stage will ease you into the right way to eat to shift the balance from inflamed to healing. A lot is going on at this stage as your body begins to return to equilibrium and repairs any damage that being unbalanced has caused. You will learn about the intensity factor needed in exercise for quick results. You should already be seeing the benefits of your relaxation practice and might want to increase your commitment. I show you what an ideal day at this stage looks like, including breakfast, lunch, dinner, snacks, supplements, exercise, and relaxation.

WEEK 4 AND AFTER: RENEW/THE NEW LIFESTYLE

Most programs would call this the "maintenance" stage, but that's too boring for me. As the changes you are working on approach becoming habits, you will be renewed. When your body is back in balance, you will feel better and better. Just as you wouldn't leave the house without brushing your teeth in the morning, eating well, moving, and handling whatever life throws your way with serenity will eventually become automatic. A week's meal plan for how to eat for the rest of your life will point you in the right direction. An adaptable workout for staying fit and strong without pushing yourself too hard will keep you moving safely. You will gain confidence in your ability to handle pressure and upsets in a positive way that does not cost you your well-being.

WHEN NEEDED: REFRESH/GETTING BACK ON

No one is perfect. A holiday, a tight deadline, layoffs at work, moving to a new home, the illness and death of a parent, there are so many things that can disrupt the routines you are trying to establish. When your stress levels rise, your body sets off an inflammatory cascade. You might revert to your old eating habits and start bingeing on sweets, chips, baked goods, and highly processed foods. And forget about exercise. You couldn't possibly squeeze in a workout. As for relaxing, you have too much on your mind to take a breath and sit still. When the demands of life seem overwhelming and you lose sight of what you have to do to stay healthy, you need to refresh your resolve to take care of yourself.

I recommend supplements to take and foods to eat to help you get back on track and manage cravings for sweets and junk food. Emergency relaxation techniques and stress-busting workouts will help you defuse tension and stimulate yourself in a healthy way. In no time at all, you will be back in control and feeling great.

The program is followed by over sixty remarkable recipes that prove that eating for balance does not have to be a hardship with bland and unexciting meals. Trying these recipes will convince you that eating well can be satisfying and a treat.

The Mouth⇔Body Connection covers new ground that is just entering public awareness. I want to deliver the good news that you can take simple steps to protect or restore your health by starting with the mouth⇔body connection.

PART I

THE MOUTH ⇔ BODY CONNECTION

Chapter One

Worlds Within

You are more microbial than human. Your body hosts 100 trillion microorganisms, which have their own genes. According to the most recent estimates, your body consists of 37 trillion human cells. **The composition of your body has three times more microorganisms than human cells.** These microbes, which consist of bacteria, fungi, viruses, protozoa, and archaea, form dynamic communities in and on your body. Wherever your body is exposed to the outside world—your skin, mouth, nasal passages, lungs, digestive and urogenital tracts—a microbial community exists. The moister the area, the denser the microbial population. The sum of these microbes and their genes constitute the human microbiome. Your microbiome is as unique as your fingerprint.

Exploring the synergistic and symbiotic relationship between man and microbes is redefining what it is to be human. Humanity is now seen as a relationship between human cells and the microbiome, the interaction forming a "superorganism." A deeper understanding of how this superorganism functions will give us more effective means of preventing disease and promoting wellness.

In 2008, the National Institutes of Health launched the Human Microbiome Project to study the communities of microbial cells that live in and on the human body and to assess their role in human health and disease. Scientists are now able to use gene sequencing to identify and analyze the microorganisms that inhabit the body. In the past, microbes had to be grown in a petri dish to identify them, which was limiting, because only about 20 percent of the microbes would grow in culture. New techniques have opened up a vast, unexplored territory. The relationship between humans and their microbiome and how the microbiome changes with disease have become the focus of groundbreaking research. **As science learns more about the microbial ecosystems that thrive in the body, our understanding of health and disease is being rewritten.**

For example, the microbiome is capable of making us genetically stronger. At birth, humans inherit a blueprint of 20,000 genes. The genes of resident microbes number around 8 million, nearly 400 genes for every human gene. These nonhuman genes supply us with a huge store of genetic capability. **The genes of the microbiome can provide resources and traits that have not evolved with our bodies.** Since the genomes of microorganisms change more rapidly than human genes, the presence of microbial genes can allow humans to adapt and thrive more quickly to changes in the environment. The microbial genetic pool is a resource that can make us stronger and better able to rise to ever-increasing challenges to our health.

FROM THE GERM THEORY TO BALANCE

The concept that bacteria were a determining factor in disease came into acceptance in the 1880s. Robert Koch, inspired by Louis Pasteur's germ theory, began to study tuberculosis. Koch and his team set out to prove that specific microbes or pathogens caused particular diseases. They demonstrated that single microorganisms caused anthrax, cholera, and tuberculosis. Koch's work had a profound effect on medicine. Identifying and studying the causes of various illnesses was a step toward preventing and curing infectious diseases. Considered the father of modern bacteriology, Koch won a Nobel Prize for his work. He assumed that disease could be attributed to a particular microbe and that disease-causing microbes were not found in healthy people. Koch's groundbreaking work launched microbiology research that took more than a hundred years to evolve to the study of the microbiome.

In the past ten years, there has been a momentous shift in our understanding of disease. Rather than looking for a single microbe that causes an illness, researchers are following a multifaceted approach based on a healthy microbial balance. Until the first phase of the Human Microbiome Project from 2007 to 2012, the abundant community of human-associated microbes had not been the focus of much research. The influence of the microbiome on human development, physiology, immunity, and nutrition was a mystery. The international project, as ambitious as the Human Genome Project, which sequenced DNA, is mapping uncharted territory. Scientists are studying the relationships between the microbial ecosystems that reside in our bodies and our human cells and systems.

Research has discovered that microorganisms that are found in healthy as well as diseased people cause some illnesses. Many potential pathogens cause disease only when the microbiome is disturbed or the microbes gain access to a part of the body where they do not normally live. The presence of a pathogen does not necessarily mean disease will develop, because the microbial community is organized to keep potentially unfriendly microbes in check. When your microbiome is balanced, a newly introduced pathogen may not cause disease. If your microbiome has been disrupted, exposure to the same pathogen might make you sick.

Many diseases now appear to result solely from a disturbance in a microbial community and not a foreign invader. Instead, disease can occur when the proportions of the microbes in a community change or the behavior of the members of the community is altered under stressful conditions. These insights represent a radically new perspective on how sickness develops. **Not only do we know that human health depends on maintaining a balanced relationship with and within complex communities of microorganisms, but microbes are recognized to contribute to disease in previously unexpected ways.**

The Mouth⇔Body Connection is concerned with the unique natural ecology of the mouth. After the gut, the oral microbiome is the most diverse community of microbes in the human body. There are 20 billion resident microbes existing in your mouth at any given time with more than 600 different microorganisms represented. Their relationship with you and one another can be commensal, when one organism benefits without affecting the other; symbiotic, when the interdependence benefits both; and pathogenic, when the microbe causes harm or illness.

The oral microbiome is very dynamic, because your mouth is continuously exposed to the external environment. As a result, the oral microbiome has evolved skills to deal with challenges that other, more protected microbial communities do not experience.

Several microhabitats coexist in your mouth—on your teeth, tongue, cheeks, gums, and hard and soft palates. The microbial community found in each habitat has a different bacterial profile. In other words, each neighborhood is different. Depending on surface structures and functions, different types of microorganisms prefer distinct locations. Each neighborhood has the best conditions and nutrients for the particular microbial community that inhabits it. Despite their differences, the communities residing in your mouth live in cooperation with one another and in a symbiotic relationship with you. The microbes create an internal architecture that facilitates nutrient absorption, waste removal, and overall survival.

Microbes are intelligent. They communicate with other microbes like them to sense population densities and adjust their growth rates to stay in balance. Planktonic organisms, which populate free-flowing saliva, differ from the organisms that adhere to the surfaces of the teeth, gums, and mucous membranes. Planktonic organisms communicate with other microbes through a process called quorum sensing, using genetic information and chemical markers to ensure that the community survives and thrives.

Biodiversity is essential for good health. Each of the hundreds of types of microbes that calls your mouth home carries out a specific function required to maintain equilibrium. These ecosystems contribute to your longevity to guarantee theirs. If your microbiome made you sick, the microorganisms would have less chance of survival themselves. Survival requires an intricate balancing act. When the community is balanced, otherwise virulent microorganisms are kept in check and can be "friendly," benign, and beneficial.

The relationship between the mouth and the rest of the body is bidirectional. Your mouth mirrors what is happening in your body. Some systemic conditions produce signs in the mouth, including increasing the severity of periodontal disease. At the same time, your mouth is the gateway to the rest of your body. I started the introduction with a long list of serious systemic conditions associated with periodontal disease. The latest research is showing that the health of your mouth has an impact on your overall health. Bacteria in your mouth can hijack your immune system and cause infection in other parts of your body. The next chapter explores how the state of your mouth can be an early warning system.

Chapter Two

A Mirror

From Your Body to Your Mouth

By now, you realize that the underlying theme of this book is that oral and general health are closely interlinked. Your mouth mirrors what is happening in the rest of your body and can provide early signs of systemic disease, because your microbiome changes when you are sick.

I often see evidence of systemic disease in a patient's mouth before a patient is aware of the condition. The mouth reflects the overall state of the body, including hydration and the health of various organs. When I shine a light in the mouths of my patients, I examine the color and pigmentation of the mucous membrane lining the mouth, look for lesions on the palate as well as the mouth's lining, evaluate the tongue, check the gums, and study the condition of tooth enamel.

Susan is a longtime patient with excellent periodontal health. Now thirty-one, she had been a patient since she was a teenager. When she came to see me for her regular quarterly checkup, her gums were inflamed and bled easily. I asked her if there had been any changes in her overall health. She said no. Then we both had an "ah-ha" moment. I knew that the rapid hormonal changes of very early pregnancy may cause sensitivity in the mouth and pregnancy gingivitis. She realized that her period was slightly late. It hadn't occurred to her that she might be pregnant. When we told each other what we were thinking, we were both delighted. She called after her positive pregnancy test to tell me that I knew before she and her husband did.

The portal to the oral cavity is your lips. They show systemic changes through their color and hydration. For example, dry, cracking lips are sometimes seen in people with diabetes. Vitamin deficiencies can cause thin, receding lips.

A change in the color of the oral membrane is a most easily identified change. A pale color can indicate anemia. Hyperpigmentation or darkening may be the first indication of adrenal insufficiency with diseases like Addison's. Chronic liver disease can turn the membrane in the area under the tongue and soft palate yellow. Changes in the color of the oral mucous membranes can be related to tobacco use, medications, and dietary insufficiencies as well. Erosion of the teeth—the wearing down of enamel—can be a symptom of gastroesophageal reflux disease (GERD). Reflux is the result of acid backing up from the stomach, which can lead to the destruction of dental enamel.

Greg, who was in his mid-thirties, came to the office for a routine examination. I found a lump, a swelling on the inside of his left cheek that was not related to saliva glands, dental problems, or an external infection of the face. I was concerned. The oral pathologist I sent him to performed a biopsy. Greg was diagnosed with non-Hodgkin's lymphoma. From his mouth, the cancer could easily have spread to the rest of his lymphatic system. Memorial Sloan Kettering made a customized chemotherapy cocktail for him, which saved his life.

To avoid bogging you down with too much medical information, I have created a table to give you an idea of where and how symptoms of systemic conditions can appear in the mouth.

Oral Symptoms of Systemic Disease

Disease	Inflammation	Tongue	Gums	Teeth	Symptoms
Diabetes mellitus	x	x			Gum bleeding, inflammation, and disease, yeast infection, smooth tongue, taste dysfunction, dry mouth, burning mouth syndrome, delayed wound healing
Anemia	x	x			Pale gum tissue and tongue, smooth tongue, yeast infection, ulcers, mucosal burning, pain, or tenderness
Addison's disease	x				Darkening gums, yeast infection
Chronic liver disease	x				Yellow pigmentation in oral cavity
Hepatitis C	x				White, lacy patches; red, swollen gum tissues; open sores that may cause burning and pain
Crohn's disease	x				Swollen gums and mucosa, ulcerated oral lesions
Ulcerative colitis		x			Canker sores inside lips or mucous membranes of the mouth where there is no attachment to bone
Sarcoidosis		x			Painless ulceration of gums, inside lips, or mucous membranes, and palate

Oral Symptoms of Systemic Disease					
Disease	*Inflammation*	*Tongue*	*Gums*	*Teeth*	*Symptoms*
Leukemia		x	x		Bleeding, enlarged gums, secondary infections like herpes or candida
HIV			x		Periodontal disease, ulcerative gingivitis, rapid loss of periodontal attachment, pain, bleeding gums, halitosis
Non-Hodgkin's lymphoma			x		Nonpainful mass that enlarges slowly, often in the area between the cheek and teeth, the hard palate, or gum tissue
Reflux disease				x	Dental erosion, burning sensation, palatal lesions, water brash (regurgitation of an excessive accumulation of saliva from the lower part of the esophagus often with some acid material from the stomach—compare heartburn) or acidic saliva.
Bulimia/Anorexia				x	Dental erosion, increased caries rate, dry mouth, swelling of the salivary glands
Stress	x			x	Teeth grinding that leads to dental erosion, mouth sores, TMD disorders involving the jaw, and gum disease

Oral Symptoms of Systemic Disease					
Disease	Inflammation	Tongue	Gums	Teeth	Symptoms
Vitamin A deficiency	x				Dryness of membranes, lips retreat, inflammation at corner of mouth
Vitamin B$_{12}$ deficiency		x			Swollen, red tongue; inflammation on corners of mouth
Vitamin B$_3$ deficiency		x			Swollen, dark red, smooth tongue

As you can see on the table of oral symptoms, **the tongue is an area in the mouth that can be a gauge of your overall health.** Both Western and Chinese medicine diagnose illness based on the color and texture of the tongue. The color of your tongue can telegraph information about your circulatory system and the levels of oxygen in your body. Tongue coating can indicate how well your digestive system is working.

In Traditional Chinese Medicine, tongue diagnosis is a very important procedure, because the tongue is considered to be the window to the health of the entire body. A Chinese medicine practitioner examines the tongue first. Different parts of the tongue correspond to different internal organs and meridians in the Chinese system. Illustration 1 shows different locations and the organs believed to be connected.

I am not going into a full discussion of Traditional Chinese Medicine. I mention this only to show that thousands of years ago the Chinese were examining the tongue and mouth for symptoms of disharmony in the body. Oral examination has been considered an important diagnostic tool for millennia. Only recently has Western science begun to recognize the connection.

Illustration 1: The Tongue as a Map of the Organs in
Traditional Chinese Medicine

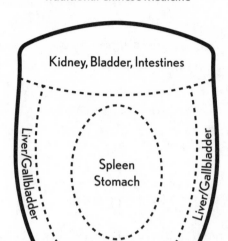

Bill, a new patient, was overweight at fifty-seven. As we reviewed his medical history, he said his gums were bleeding more than usual. When I examined his mouth, I found inflamed gums and signs of recurrent and new tooth decay. We reviewed his medical history. He told me he was working under extreme stress. He couldn't get enough to drink, and he had developed strong food cravings. During our time together, he had to leave the dental chair twice to use the restroom. The symptoms were classic.

I sent him to a doctor, who found that Bill had type 2 diabetes. Poorly controlled diabetes increases the risk and severity of oral disease, and the rate of periodontal bone loss. Consistently high blood sugar can lead to a chronic inflammatory-immune response. The excess inflammatory substances make their way into the tissues that support the teeth, where they can loosen teeth, form pockets, and cause other oral complications, such as burning mouth syndrome, fungal infections, tooth decay, and salivary functional disorders.

A healthy tongue is pink and is covered with small papillae or nodules. Allowing you to talk, swallow, and taste food, your tongue is in constant use. If you experience a change in its normal appearance or soreness, you will notice, because tongue problems can be annoying and uncomfortable. Most problems will resolve quickly, but you should get medical advice if discoloration or pain lasts more than two weeks. Your tongue can be sending you warning signals. Let's take a look at some of those symptoms and what causes them.

WHITE COATING OR PATCHES

If your tongue has a lumpy white coating the consistency of cottage cheese, you could have an oral yeast infection known as candidiasis or thrush. This condition can occur in people who have diabetes that is not well controlled, who are taking inhaled steroids for asthma or lung disease, who are on chemotherapy, or who have weakened immune systems. Oral thrush is likely to develop after the use of antibiotics, because antibiotics can kill off bacteria and allow yeast, which is not affected by antibiotics, to take over.

White patches on your tongue can be a symptom of **leukoplakia**, caused by excessive growth of cells in the mouth. Leukoplakia can develop when the tongue has been irritated. I often see it in patients who smoke. The patches can also be produced by the abrasion of a tooth rubbing against the tongue. The condition is not dangerous, but it can be a precursor to cancer, especially if you smoke. White patches on your tongue should send you to your dentist to find out what is causing the condition. A biopsy might be necessary.

Oral **lichen planus** consists of a network of raised white, lacey lines on the tongue. The condition usually heals on its own. My advice to my patients who develop a lacey tongue is to avoid smoking and limit eating foods that can cause irritation in the mouth, especially acidic foods, which you will learn about in Chapter 7.

STRAWBERRY OR RED TONGUE

A number of conditions can cause the tongue to turn red. In some cases, the texture can be smooth and glossy. In others, the tongue looks like a strawberry with enlarged taste buds dotting the surface. If you have a high fever and a red tongue, contact a doctor immediately. You could have **scarlet fever** and require antibiotics. If a child under the age of five develops a red tongue, redness and swelling in the hands and feet, and has a high fever, take the child to a doctor immediately. It could be **Kawasaki syndrome**, a rare autoimmune disease that affects the blood vessels.

Vitamin B$_{12}$ and iron deficiencies may turn your tongue red. Vitamin B$_{12}$ and iron are needed for papillae on the tongue to mature. If you are deficient in those two nutrients, you lose papillae, and your tongue takes on a smooth appearance. Vegetarians are prone to have low levels of B$_{12}$, which is found in meat. Supplements are needed to make up the deficiency.

When reddish spots appear on your tongue, you probably have a common condition called **geographic tongue**, because the pattern of the red spots can look like a map. The patches are sometimes bordered in white and their positions on the tongue may shift. If the patches persist for more than two weeks, have your dentist take a look at your mouth to make sure the redness is actually geographic tongue, which is usually harmless. If your tongue feels sore, your doctor might prescribe an anti-inflammatory topical or antihistamine rinse.

BLACK, HAIRY TONGUE

This condition sounds much worse than it is, but it can be alarming. The papillae on the surface of your tongue are always growing.

Though chewing, drinking, and talking usually wear them down, papillae may grow long for some people. Excessively long papillae provide a harbor for bacteria, which grow and look black. These overgrown papillae take on the appearance of hair. Smoking or drinking coffee or dark teas can contribute to the darkening. If you practice good oral hygiene, you are not likely to develop a black, hairy tongue. People who are diabetic, on antibiotics, or chemotherapy are more likely to develop the condition. Using a tongue scraper or brushing the tongue may be enough to solve the problem.

CRACKS AND CREVICES

Your tongue shows signs of aging, too, and wrinkling and cracks are not uncommon. Poor-fitting dentures can cause indentations on the sides of the tongue. Problems may arise if fungal infections develop inside the crevices, causing a bad odor, pain, and burning. Infections are treated with a topical antifungal medication. Drink plenty of water and brush your tongue if you have fissures on your tongue.

SORE, BUMPY TONGUE

Many factors may contribute to a sore, bumpy tongue, including:

- **Trauma.** Scalding your tongue with hot food or beverages can be painful until the tongue heals. Clenching or grinding your teeth can be irritating to the sides of the tongue.
- **Enlarged papillae.** Papillae that become infected or irritated and enlarged can be painful, especially when you eat and drink. Many conditions and actions cause enlarged, painful papillae. The chemicals that enter your mouth when you smoke cigarettes irritate the tongue, resulting

in sore, enlarged papillae. Gastrointestinal issues can contribute to this problem. GERD and ulcerative colitis are known to cause the condition. Stress is involved in the development of enlarged papillae. Finally, enlarged papillae could be a sign of oral cancer. If symptoms of swollen papillae worsen or do not improve in a few weeks, consult a medical professional.

- **Canker sores.** These sores occur on the tongue and the lining of the mouth. After four or five days, the pain subsides and the ulcers should disappear within two weeks. The cause of canker sores is not known, but the odds are that it is something viral. Canker sores are associated with stress, and often appear when people are run down. Do not confuse a canker sore with a cold sore, which usually appears on the lips. A cold sore, which is caused by the herpes simplex virus, is extremely contagious. Symptoms of diabetes and anemia include a sore tongue.

- **Oral cancer.** Consult with your doctor if a sore or lump on your tongue is not gone in a week or two. Be aware that many early-stage oral cancers are not painful. Do not assume that you are fine if a sore or bump does not hurt.

BURNING TONGUE SYNDROME

Women are seven times more likely than men to develop this condition, which affects up to 15 percent of the population. Post-menopausal women in particular are more likely to suffer from this syndrome. Though the tongue looks normal, hormonal changes may cause a stinging and burning sensation, as if the tongue had been scalded. The mouth may feel dry and thirst increases. Taste may change and become bitter or metallic or taste might be lost entirely. The discomfort has many different patterns and can come and go.

Now that you have an understanding of how the mouth serves as a mirror reflecting the internal state of your body, let's look at the other side of this bidirectional relationship. As the gateway to the body, your mouth can act as an *agent provocateur* for systemic disease.

Chapter Three

The Gateway

From Your Mouth to Your Body

Before exploring the mouth as a gateway to the rest of the body and the effects of gum disease on systemic illness, I would like to mention three conditions that appear to be bidirectional, namely diabetes, obesity, and osteoporosis. **Dynamic, two-way relationships between the oral microbiome and the body demonstrate how complex the interactions are.**

DIABETES GOES BOTH WAYS

Diabetes has reached epidemic proportions. The Centers for Disease Control and Prevention reported in 2015 that 29.1 million people, or 9.3 percent of the U.S. population, have diabetes. Of that number, 8.1 million people are undiagnosed. In adults twenty and older, more than one in every ten people suffers from diabetes, and in people sixty-five and older, that figure rises to more than one in four. The global statistics are as alarming. The number of adults with type 2 or adult-onset diabetes is projected to rise from 171 million in 2000 to 366 million in 2030. The mouth may present one way to curb this disease.

The strong link between diabetes and periodontal disease goes from the mouth to the body as well as from body to mouth. You have seen how diabetes manifests in the mouth in the table on page 18, but an unhealthy mouth may contribute to developing diabetes or worsening the condition. In other words, **having diabetes increases the risk for periodontitis, and gum inflammation negatively affects glycemic control, which is at the core of diabetes.** The bacteria involved in oral disease interfere with the body's ability to regulate the amount of glucose circulating in the bloodstream. When too much glucose is present, the pancreas pumps out insulin, which functions to help cells absorb glucose and store the energy. As insulin levels rise, the hormone stops working effectively, and the cells resist absorbing glucose. Insulin resistance leads to high levels of blood sugar, which may develop into diabetes. Bacteria from the oral microbiome can directly contribute to rising blood sugar levels that can produce insulin resistance and diabetes.

OBESITY AS A VICIOUS CYCLE

Obesity is another example of bidirectionality in the mouth⇔ body connection. In the past, obesity was considered a problem of willpower, involving the consumption of too many sweets and high-calorie foods. We now know that the source of the problem is systemic. Fat cells secrete particular types of pro-inflammatory cytokines and hormones that trigger inflammation. The more fat you have, the more likely your body is to be inflamed. **Many studies have shown that being overweight is associated with greater risk of periodontal disease and tooth loss.** I often find yeast infections in the mouths of people who are significantly overweight. Researchers have assumed that periodontal disease in overweight people develops from high levels of internal inflammation.

Rachel, who was obese, came to see me before attempting to get pregnant a second time. She had had her first baby before she was a patient. Her baby boy was premature, born at thirty-five weeks weighing four and a half pounds. He spent a couple of weeks in an incubator in neonatal intensive care. She had done a lot of reading and learned there was a connection between obesity and gum disease and gum disease and preterm, low-birth-weight babies. She definitely did not want to go through that again. She was determined to resolve any issues in her mouth before becoming pregnant.

On examination, I found her tongue had a white coating and her mouth was very yeasty. She also had low-grade gum disease. We scheduled treatments for her gums, and I gave her my diet plan to fight inflammation. Determined to reduce inflammation, she had periodontal work done on her teeth with antibiotic injections. She followed my Triple A Diet and began to lose weight. She continued on the Curatola Care Program for six months, until she was ready to get pregnant.

She is in her last month of pregnancy as I write this, and her sonograms show a robust baby of normal weight.

One team of scientists has asked the question, "Is obesity an oral bacterial disease?" They speculate that weight gain could be the result of a change in the oral microbiome. They found that of the forty species of bacteria they surveyed in groups of overweight and healthy-weight women, significant differences were present in the saliva of the overweight group in seven of the forty species they studied. More than 98 percent of the overweight women could be identified by the presence of a single bacterial species, *S. noxia*. This bacterium, which is also found in the gut, is anaerobic, one of the bad guys that takes over when the oral microbiome is disrupted. It appears likely that an excess of this bacterium in the mouth could indicate a developing overweight condition and possibly be responsible for weight gain.

The relationship between obesity and oral bacteria is complex. Though the research is preliminary, I mention the study because it captures the exciting potential of what the research on the microbiome is on the verge of discovering. I hope that by the time the book is published, I will be able to report on a new contributing factor to the obesity epidemic.

OSTEOPOROSIS

Periodontal disease and osteoporosis both involve bone loss. Osteoporosis and periodontitis share risk factors, including age, smoking, and estrogen deficiency. Osteopenia, an early stage of osteoporosis, results when bone resorption is higher than bone formation. The resulting demineralization leads to full-blown osteoporosis. This disorder compromises bone strength, which increases the risk of fracture. In women, estrogen deficiency contributes to bone loss, because the hormone directly or indirectly affects cytokines that help to regulate bone metabolism as well as the inflammatory response. Osteoporosis is a risk factor for periodontal disease. The systemic inflammation in the body can affect bone loss in the mouth.

Periodontal disease is characterized by the resorption of bone and the loss of soft tissue attachment of the teeth. Excessive resorption can be an effect of chronic inflammation in the mouth. Studies have found that the gram-negative bacteria found in periodontal disease can trigger resorption in the rest of the body. To date, scientists do not know which comes first or if it varies from case to case. Though the relationship between periodontal disease and osteoporosis needs further clarification, there is undeniably a connection.

THE MOUTH AS A GATEWAY

The oral microbiome is an open system exposed to the environment. The possibility of foreign invaders entering your body from your mouth is heightened, because your oral microbiome is in contact with foods, liquids, and air, all of which may contain pathogens and toxins. Bacteria from your mouth can enter your bloodstream through small abrasions caused by trauma due to eating, brushing, flossing, biting the tongue or lips, or even using toothpicks. Bacteria may be aspirated into the respiratory system, leading to pulmonary infections like pneumonia.

Since the mouth is a significant entryway, microorganisms that inhabit that area can spread to other parts of your body. Pathogens living in your mouth can pass through mucous membranes and pockets formed by gum disease and enter your bloodstream. The inflammatory response caused by periodontal disease can complicate already existing chronic conditions. Infections in the mouth often involve anaerobic bacteria, which are not dependent on air and thrive in the deep pockets caused by periodontal disease.

ONE OF THE BAD GUYS

Fusobacterium nucleatum is a gram-negative, anaerobic oral bacterium that can live in the mouth without causing problems or can behave as a pathogen that is associated with a wide spectrum of diseases. Though there are hundreds of species of bacteria living in your mouth, focusing on one will explain the mouth to body dynamic in disease. This previously overlooked microorganism has been discovered to play an important role in disease.

F. nucleatum is abundant in the oral microbiome and absent or rarely detected elsewhere in the body under normal conditions. Under disease conditions, *F. nucleatum* is one of the most prevalent microbes found in sites outside of the mouth. This one species of bacteria, with five identified subspecies, has been associated with the following diseases:

- **Oral infections:** chronic periodontitis, aggressive periodontitis, gingivitis, endodontic infections.
- **Adverse pregnancy outcomes:** chorioamnionitis, an inflammation of the fetal membranes; preterm birth; stillbirth;

neonatal sepsis; preeclampsia, a pregnancy complication involving high blood pressure.

* **Gastrointestinal disorders:** Colorectal cancer, inflammatory bowel disease, appendicitis.
* **Other infections:** Atherosclerosis, cerebral aneurysm, COPD, other respiratory tract infections, organ abscesses, rheumatoid arthritis, Alzheimer's disease.

F. nucleatum has been detected in denser quantities in the saliva of patients with gingivitis and periodontitis compared to those without oral disease. The prevalence of the microbe increases with the severity of the gum disease and the progression of inflammation.

As you'll remember from Susan's case history, pregnancy gingivitis is common. *F. nucleatum* is the most prevalent oral microorganism found in amniotic fluid and cord blood in adverse pregnancy outcomes. Finding the bacterium outside the mouth demonstrates its ability to spread. This bacterium has been detected in placental and fetal tissues, including amniotic fluid, fetal membranes, cord blood, and fetal lung and stomach. *F. nucleatum* has been the predominant microbe found in amniotic fluid and fetal membrane in preterm births.

This bacterium has only recently been linked to colorectal cancer, but the connection has already generated many studies. It has been found in colorectal tumors along with other oral microorganisms. Irritable bowel disease is a risk factor for colorectal cancer, so it is not surprising that the same microorganisms are involved in both diseases. Strains of the bacterium that have been isolated from the inflamed tissues of irritable bowel syndrome patients are more invasive than those from normal tissues.

F. nucleatum is often detected in the atherosclerotic plaques of patients with cardiovascular disease, and is one of the most common periodontal pathogens found in ruptured cerebral aneurysms. Periodontal treatment has also been shown to improve rheumatoid arthritis.

I have concentrated on this one pathogenic microbe to give you a sense of how much trouble oral bacteria can cause in the rest of the body.

INFLAMMATION 101

Understanding the process of inflammation is the foundation for explaining the mouth⇔body connection. Though inflammation is commonly considered a bad thing, you could not survive without it. **Inflammation is a protective response to get rid of whatever causes injury to cells and to stop the consequences of the injury.** Trauma, genetic defects, toxic physical and chemical agents, foreign bodies, immune reactions, and infections, all can be damaging. Their presence excites the immune system, and inflammation results.

Inflammation is either acute or chronic. Acute inflammation has a rapid onset and short duration. Chronic inflammation is prolonged and puts the healing process into overdrive.

Bacteria trigger the production of inflammatory mediators to direct the response. When these mediators are present in the body for extended periods of time, they can be harmful.

The most graphic way to describe the process is to compare it to a battle. When a harmful organism invades the body, the immune system rallies to attack and destroy it. Many types of invasions can trigger the immune system, which fights back with inflammation to defend your body from harm. Inflammation can be caused by pathogens—bacteria, viruses, or fungi—external injuries such as cuts, foreign objects such as a splinter, or the effects of chemicals or radiation.

When an invading organism threatens to damage tissue, substances from the tissue called antigens alert immune cells to race to the site of the attack. Many different immune cells join the fray. Hormones such as histamine produced by the tissue cause the blood vessels in the affected tissue to expand, which allows more blood to reach the battlefield. That is why the inflamed area turns red and becomes hot. Depending on the site of the battlefield and the type of invader, the initial defense of the immune system to an infection varies. The cells of the immune system communicate and cooperate in a complex way. Here is an overview of immune system warriors:

- The invader most often is recognized by **lymphocytes**, white blood cells that determine the appropriate immune response.
- The lungs and intestines are primarily defended by **macrophages**, which means "big eaters" in Greek. The first cells of the immune system on the scene begin to digest the invading organism. Proteins from the destroyed bacteria, called antigens, stimulate other immune system cells into action.
- Some bacteria, including *Staphylococcus aureus* and *Salmonella Typhi*, produce substances called chemotaxins, which arouse the immune system. The chemotaxins activate immune cells called **phagocytes**, which destroy the invaders.
- Other bacteria are recognized by a system that sounds the alarm by producing chemical messengers called **cytokines**, which activate phagocytes. The invading bacteria are marked with chemicals that make them stand out. In the process, chemicals are released, which promote the inflammatory response.

As you can see, this complex battle plan enlists an army of soldiers. Each of the actions I have just described stimulates the phagocytes to move to the site of the invasion. When the phagocytes begin to digest and destroy the invading bacteria, they produce more cytokines, which activate even more immune cells. The initial immune reaction leads to a cascade of reactions.

The first physical effect of an acute inflammatory response is for blood circulation to increase at the site of the invasion. Blood vessels located near the battlefield, the site of the invasion, dilate to send troops to the area by increasing blood flow. Gaps open in the cell walls that surround the infected area to allow the immune cells to pass from the blood. Increased blood flow means a stronger immune response.

An army of different immune cells congregates at the site of the inflammation along with a supply of ammunition, proteins that fuel the immune response. This produces an increase in body heat, which in itself can have an antibiotic effect that swings the balance of chemical reactions in favor of the healthy cells. The tissue in the affected area becomes red and warm as a result of all the blood that has reached the site. The tissue becomes swollen for the same reason. The area can become painful, because the tissues have expanded, which can cause pressure on nerve cells.

The war usually continues until the infection has been eradicated. Pus is the debris left over from the immune battle. The process shuts off once the threat of infection has passed. If the foreign antigen is not eradicated, or if the immune cells receive a stay-alive signal, chronic inflammation may develop. With chronic inflammation, the immune soldiers that are capable of destroying microbes can cause collateral damage.

Sometimes the immune system receives a faulty distress signal and deploys an unnecessary Special Forces squad. Those immune soldiers still mobilize even though a threat is not present. Since there is no infection for them to attack, they remain deployed, often for a long time. Your body is not equipped to handle unfocused immune activity. Eventually, those immune warriors may start damaging your internal organs.

With chronic inflammation, your body is always on high alert. A prolonged state of emergency can damage your brain, heart, and other organs. For example, when inflammatory cells remain active in blood vessels, they may promote the accumulation of plaque, which is made of cholesterol, fatty substances, cellular waste products, calcium, and fibrin, a clotting material in the blood. The body reacts to this plaque as foreign and sends more of its first responders. As the plaque continues to build, the arteries can thicken, causing hardening of the arteries or atherosclerosis, which raises the risk of heart attack or stroke.

Recent research has shown that inflammation in the brain may play a role in Alzheimer's disease. The brain was formerly considered off-limits to inflammation because of the blood-brain barrier—a built-in security system that does not allow certain substances to enter the brain. Scientists have now demonstrated, however, that immune cells can and do infiltrate the brain during times of distress. I will discuss the association between gum disease and Alzheimer's disease in more detail later in this chapter.

This introduction to the process of inflammation explains how chronic inflammation can lead to disease. Now we are ready to focus in on the connection between the mouth and systemic illness.

PATHS TO SYSTEMIC ILLNESS

Only recently has gum disease been seen to originate or affect the course of a growing number of systemic diseases, including cardiovascular disease, bacterial pneumonia and other pulmonary diseases, diabetes, and fetal development. Scientists are studying three pathways that link oral infections to systemic disease:

Pathway 1
Infection can spread from the oral cavity because of bacteria that travel to other locations in the body. **Oral infections and dental procedures can allow microbes to gain entrance to the blood and circulate throughout the body.** Usually these microorganisms are eliminated within minutes and do not cause

problems, but if the traveling microbes find favorable conditions, they might settle in and begin to multiply.

Systemic diseases associated with Pathway 1:

- Bacterial infections may produce growths on the cells lining the inside of the heart, known as the endocardium.
- Inflammation of the heart.
- Brain abscesses, inflamed collections of pus, immune cells, and other material.
- A blood clot within a sinus cavity at the base of the brain.
- Inflammation of sinuses.
- Inflammation of the eye.
- Skin ulcers.
- Infection of the bones.
- Infection in a replaced joint, which is why people who have had joint replacement surgery have to take antibiotics before dental work.

Pathway 2

The microbes involved in gum infections can produce toxins that affect the rest of the body. I will go into this in more detail in the next chapter. For now, it is sufficient to know that, when balance is disrupted, "bad guy" microbes produce toxins that are lethal poisons. These oral microbial toxins damage the body and contribute to many illnesses.

Systemic diseases associated with Pathway 2:

- Stroke caused by a blockage in the blood vessels that supply blood to the brain.
- Heart attack resulting from the blockage of one or more coronary arteries.

- Abnormal pregnancy outcomes such as low birth weight and prematurity.
- Chronic fever, a low-grade fever than lasts longer than ten to fourteen days.
- Facial pain, either brief, electric-shock-like pain or a less intense, dull, burning pain caused by inflammation of the fifth cranial nerve.
- Toxic shock syndrome, a life-threatening complication of certain bacterial infections, experienced most commonly in women.
- Immunodeficiency, a malfunction of the immune system.
- Chronic meningitis, inflammation of the protective layers of the brain and spinal cord that lasts four weeks or more.

Pathway 3
Oral microorganisms can trigger an immune response that causes inflammation throughout the body. When an antigen, a molecule perceived as a harmful, foreign entity, enters the bloodstream, it causes an immune response that creates antibodies to neutralize the antigen. When the pathogen reacts with an antibody, they form an immune complex. These combinations of antigens and antibodies give rise to various acute and chronic inflammatory reactions.

Systemic diseases associated with Pathway 3:

- Inflamed blood vessels throughout the body.
- Chronic hives that last six weeks or more or recur often.
- Inflammation of the middle layer of the eye, which contains the pigment.
- Inflammatory bowel disease, chronic inflammation of all or part of the digestive tract.

- Ulcerative colitis, inflammation of the colon.
- Crohn's disease, chronic inflammation, usually located at the end of the small bowel, the beginning of the colon.

About four years ago, when I examined Larry, who was in his late fifties, I found severe gum disease. A high-level corporate executive, he was a very busy man. He kept putting off treatment for his periodontitis and finally did nothing about it.

He returned to my office to be checked, because he needed me to sign off before he could have open-heart surgery. I restrained myself from commenting that not taking care of his oral hygiene might well have been a contributing factor to his heart condition.

Larry was furious when I told him that he was in no shape to have the surgery. He had to take care of his gum disease before the operation would be safe for him. He complained that he had arranged to take a month off, which had not been easy. He wanted to go ahead with the surgery and take care of his oral disease afterward.

I told him he would be playing Russian roulette with five bullets in the chamber. Not only would having surgery without healing his oral disease first prolong his recuperation significantly, but also more important, he would be putting his life at risk. I refused to clear him for the surgery, which was scheduled a few days later. He stormed out of the office, and I have never seen him again.

Since then I have wondered whether his surgeon took the condition of his patient's mouth seriously. There is such a gap between the new research on oral health and how medicine is now being practiced. Everyone involved seemed to consider the oral examination a rubber stamp procedure, a formality to get out of the way. Without a doubt, that lack of awareness will soon change.

CARDIOVASCULAR DISEASE (CVD)

After adjustments for other risk factors, studies indicate that severe periodontal disease is associated with a 25 to 90 percent increase in the risk for cardiovascular disease. One study showed that 66 percent of heart-healthy patients had periodontitis while 91 percent of CVD patients had moderate to severe periodontitis. Oral bacterial DNA has been found in plaque located in the carotid, coronary, and aortic arteries.

The presence of microbes from the oral microbiome can lead to problems in two ways: Harmful bacteria can invade the arterial wall or cause the release of systemic inflammatory substances that can damage the blood vessels.

CANCER

The association between periodontal disease and cancer has been the subject of many studies. A Harvard University School of Public Health study published in 2007 uncovered a strong correlation between advanced gum disease in men to a 63 percent higher incidence of pancreatic cancer.

A British and American research team at the Imperial College in London studied the statistical health records of 50,000 men from data collected during a period of twenty-one years. They found that the presence of moderate gum disease contributed to an overall 14 percent increased risk of cancer, including lung, kidney, and blood cancers in smokers and nonsmokers. **They found a 33 percent increase in the risk of lung cancer, 50 percent rise in the risk of kidney cancer, and a 30 percent higher risk of blood cancers such as leukemia among the subjects with gum disease.** Chronic advanced gum disease had a fourfold increased risk in head and neck cancers for each millimeter of related bone loss around teeth. This study has generated extensive ongoing research on the cause of the correlation.

AGING AND ALZHEIMER'S DISEASE

Your microbiome influences how well you age. As you get older, the bacterial load in your body increases. Studies have shown that aging favors the overgrowth of oral anaerobes. This shift contributes to the rise of circulating, pro-inflammatory cytokines in your bloodstream, which can lead to a chronic state of inflammation.

I've been intrigued by studies that have just been published that link the oral microbiome, aging, and Alzheimer's disease. Prolonged exposure to high levels of circulating cytokines can compromise the integrity of the blood-brain barrier, which protects the brain from exposure to damaging substances. **When inflammation weakens the blood-brain barrier, harmful bacteria manage to pass through and can intensify the inflammatory process in the brain.** Over a period of time, the continued release of pro-inflammatory cytokines exacerbates neuronal damage in the brain, which can lead to Alzheimer's disease. Systemic inflammation is also associated with confusion in the elderly.

ADVERSE PREGNANCY OUTCOMES

Changes in hormone levels during pregnancy can influence the health of gums by promoting inflammation, which is called pregnancy gingivitis. You read about this condition with Susan's story in the previous chapter. Growing evidence that infections nowhere near the placenta and fetus may have a role in premature delivery and low-birth-weight infants has brought attention to the role of chronic bacterial infections in the body. Preterm birth is considered to be less than thirty-seven weeks of gestation, and low birth weight is less than five pounds eight ounces. Many risk factors may affect a short gestational period, including smoking, consuming alcohol, poor prenatal care, poor maternal nutrition, and urinary tract infection.

Recently, *F. nucleatum*, a bad guy pathogen, gram-negative bacterium found in the mouth, which you read about above, was isolated from the amniotic fluid, placenta, and fetal membranes of women who delivered prematurely. The pro-inflammatory cytokines the body generates in the presence of these bacteria appear to be the key mechanism linking periodontal disease to premature, low-birth-weight births. Several studies have found that soluble pro-inflammatory markers crossed the placental barrier and caused fetal toxicity that led to preterm birth.

If you are even thinking of becoming pregnant, make sure to see your dentist right away. The health of your gums can affect your pregnancy. As you focus on eating the right food and vitamins, avoiding toxins, and relaxing, do not forget the importance of your oral health. You should observe a pregnancy regimen to provide a healthy home in which your baby can grow. Just do not forget the mouth⇔body connection as you take care of yourself.

ORAL HPV (HUMAN PAPILLOMAVIRUS) INFECTION AND THROAT CANCER

HPV is a group of viruses that includes more than a hundred different strains. HPV is most commonly attributed to causing cervical cancer and genital warts, but it has been shown to cause oral cancer as well. Oral HPV infection can be divided into two types. The low-risk types cause benign cancers and warts in the mouth, while the high-risk HPV types can cause throat cancers.

Researchers from the University of Texas Health Sciences Center analyzed health statistics collected by the Centers for Disease Control and Prevention and published their study in the journal *Cancer Prevention Research*. They found that oral HPV infections lead to throat cancer and can be linked to poor oral health.

Their findings showed that the participants who reported bad oral health had a 56 percent higher risk of developing oral HPV infection compared with those who had good oral health. Those with gum disease showed a 51 percent higher risk of oral HPV infection, and dental problems led to a 28 percent higher risk. According to the researchers, **oral HPV infection causes 40 to 80 percent of all throat cancers**. One strain of HPV has been linked to a third of all throat cancers.

The researchers report that HPV needs a wound in the mouth to enter and infect oral cavities. Bad oral health could create an entryway for HPV through mouth ulcers, mucosal disruption, and chronic inflammation.

One out of two sexually active teenage girls has contracted at least one type of genital HPV infection. Throughout the course of their lives, about 75 to 89 percent of the people in the United States will contract one or more types of HPV. A vaccine was introduced about ten years ago to combat HPV, which has already reduced the virus's prevalence in teenage girls by almost two-thirds. Immunization rates remain low—about 40 percent of girls and 20 percent of boys between the ages of thirteen and seventeen. There has been resistance to the vaccine, because people associate it with adolescent sexual activity rather than cancer prevention. Efforts are being made to shift the focus of this very effective vaccine's purpose. We have the means to close the gateway from which oral HPV spreads to promote throat cancer.

Now that you know about the direct connection between your mouth and systemic illnesses, you should be convinced that your oral health matters. **Chronic, low-grade gum disease is an early warning signal that often slips beneath the radar.** Since gum disease is slow to progress and doesn't involve pain, it's easy to ignore. If your scalp bled when you brushed your hair, you would be concerned. Most people dismiss bleeding gums when they should pay attention. What seems like a minor annoyance could be a threat to your health.

The next chapter focuses on what happens when the communities in the oral microbiome become disrupted and how gum disease develops. When you know what you are up against, it is easier to take practical steps to protect yourself. Awareness creates motivation, and motivation fuels action.

Chapter Four

When Balance Is Disrupted

The oral microbiome contains more than 700 species of microbes, anywhere from 6 to 10 billion, most of which are bacteria. The mouth's microbiome is composed of:

- Water
- Salivary proteins
- Crevicular fluid, which fights inflammation and cleans waste material from the crevices between teeth and gums
- Immune complexes
- Minerals
- 6 to 10 billion microorganisms, the majority of which are bacteria

The ecosystems in your mouth are referred to as the oral biofilm.

Bacteria colonize on the hard surfaces of your teeth and the soft tissue lining your mouth. Your teeth, the space between your teeth and gums, known as the gingival sulcus, your tongue, cheeks, hard and soft palates, and tonsils provide rich environments in which microbial communities flourish. Each location has a different microbial profile.

The oral biofilm interacts with the saliva in the mouth and

the tissues below, protecting the hard tissues from drying out. In addition, the oral microbiome keeps the lining of the mouth well lubricated. The muco-proteins in saliva function like oil in a machine, and the bacteria are minute ball bearings that reduce friction as food passes by.

The microorganisms that live in your mouth adapt to changing environments by creating complex colonies. Though these communities play vital roles in maintaining oral health, they can promote disease. This chapter will show you how a protective biofilm can turn harmful.

THE MAKING OF A COMMUNITY

Biofilms are found everywhere in nature. If you have ever slipped on a rock as you were crossing a brook, you have encountered a biofilm. Wherever you find a combination of moisture, nutrients, and a surface, you are likely to find biofilm. A biofilm forms when bacteria adhere to surfaces in moist environments by excreting a slimy, sticky substance.

The five major biofilms in and on the human body are the gut, mouth, respiratory, skin, and genito-urinary. By 2002, these bacterial communities or biofilms were renamed the *microbiome* by the Nobel laureate biologist Dr. Joshua Lederberg. He described a microbial biome as being "the collective genome of our indigenous microbes (microflora)." He presented the idea that "a comprehensive genetic view of Homo Sapiens as a life-form should include the genes on our microbiome." In other words, we are a composite of species, man and microbe.

The mouth is continuously bathed with saliva that keeps conditions warm and moist at a neutral pH between 6.75 and 7.25, neither acidic nor alkaline. Saliva creates the right climate for microbial communities to thrive in your mouth. Saliva helps to maintain balance in the mouth and defends against disease. Saliva provides nutrients that protect tooth enamel and antibodies that defend the oral cavity and the rest of the body from infection.

In a balanced oral microbiome, most of the bacteria are aerobic, which means they rely on oxygen to live. In order for the aerobes to stay healthy, the biofilm needs to be structured so that molecular oxygen can reach the microbes.

Bacteria exist in two different states in your mouth: free floating and attached. Planktonic bacteria, which researchers have focused on for several decades, float solo in saliva. Further research has shown that planktonic bacteria do not stay long in this state. Saliva transports the single microbes until they find a home in the mouth, a place to settle. They can adhere to a surface or to one another.

Microorganisms seek to join a community in an attached biofilm, where there is strength in numbers. Communities of bacteria have capacities and survival strategies that exceed what an individual microorganism can do on its own. More than 99 percent of all bacteria on earth live attached.

Biofilm communities can develop in hours. Oral biofilms develop when glycoproteins from saliva coat the teeth and gums to create a salivary pellicle, a nonbacterial film, which forms rapidly after teeth are cleaned. Oral bacteria attach to the pellicle to construct the microcolonies of a biofilm. The colonies develop in five stages.

1. Initial Attachment

   A thin, bacteria-free layer called a pellicle forms on a tooth surface within minutes of cleaning. When planktonic bacteria come upon this moist surface, they can attach themselves. The process of attachment changes the genes of free-floating planktonic bacteria. The first colonists have a weak attachment to the surface.

2. Irreversible Attachment

   The microbes begin to produce a slimy substance to anchor themselves more permanently.

3. Colonization

   The biofilm grows mostly by cell division, rather than recruitment. Some species of bacteria are not able to attach

Illustration 2: Development of a biofilm community

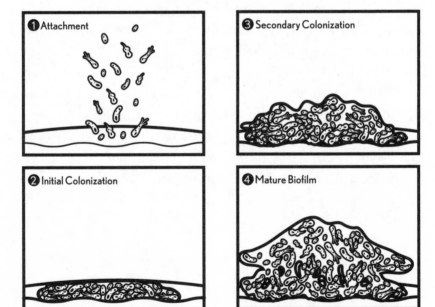

to a surface on their own but are able to anchor themselves to earlier colonists. At this stage, the colony begins to grow away from the tooth.

4. Maturation

The bacteria cluster to form mushroom-shaped colonies, which are held together by sugary molecular strands produced by the microbes. The biofilm can be as thin as a few cells.

5. Dispersal

This is an essential stage of the life cycle of the biofilm. Colonies can propagate by detaching clumps of cells or even by releasing individual cells. The detached bacteria can then attach to a surface of another biofilm or colonize new surfaces.

The structure of the biofilm provides customized living environments with differing pHs and nutrient and oxygen availability for the diverse community. A number of fluid channels allow

Illustration 3: The structure of the mature oral microbiome

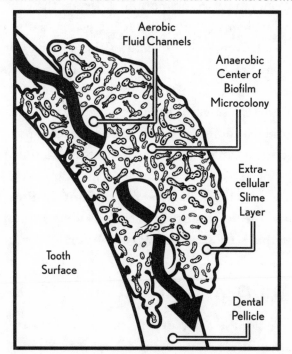

nutrients and oxygen to reach the members of the community and allow the removal of bacterial waste products. Oxygen supports aerobic bugs and keeps anaerobic bugs from overgrowing. Bacteria in the center of a colony may live in an environment without oxygen, while microbes at the edges of the fluid channels are more likely to be aerobic. The first colonizers of an oral microfilm tend to be gram-positive aerobes, which need oxygen, and facultative anaerobes, which can live with or without oxygen.

The colony builds a defense with a slime layer to protect the mushroom-shaped community from antibiotics, antimicrobials, and the body's own defense mechanisms.

The many different kinds of microbes living together in the community all get along. Each independent microcolony has its own living arrangements. The microorganisms cooperate with one another by means of several kinds of intelligence. Earlier, I mentioned quorum sensing, a mechanism that allows microbes to sense the number of their own species as well as the number of other species in a specific biofilm. They are then able to adjust their own biochemical processes to fit better in the collective. They form relatively stable structures that provide for adequate nutrition, waste removal, and community survival. Chemical signals create a system of communication among colonies.

The microorganisms can change their position within a microcolony to defend the community from a challenge or a threat, as if they were executing a battle plan. A topically applied antimicrobial substance will be met by a layer of organisms most able to prevent penetration of the microfilm. **The oral microbiome is like a meadow with many species living in harmony, but it is also like a beehive with a structure and agreed-upon job descriptions.**

WHEN THE ORAL MICROBIOME LOSES BALANCE

Another term for the oral biofilm is plaque. As you have just read, the formation of plaque is a normal process. Plaque helps with the exchange of minerals such as calcium and phosphorous and molecular oxygen. Dental plaque forms as layers on the surfaces of teeth. The proteins, minerals, and antimicrobial enzymes found in saliva control excessive plaque buildup.

If plaque builds up and hardens on your teeth, it becomes tartar or calculus, the substance that gets scraped away when you have a cleaning at your dentist's office. A thick biofilm mineralizes as saliva pumps out calcium and phosphate minerals.

Dental plaque is not the enemy when the environment in your mouth is balanced. Plaque can entrap and prevent pathogens from thriving in your mouth. On the other hand, plaque can provide refuge for a pathogen to hide from salivary flow and the immune system. Under healthy conditions, a balance between the composition of the microbes and the division of labor keeps biofilms stable.

Illustration 4 shows from left to right what happens when a microfilm loses balance.

Illustration 4: When a microbiome loses balance

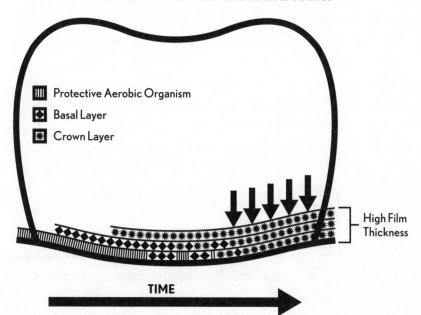

We start with a healthy microbiome, an odorless, thin film. The film is composed of mostly aerobic bacteria, which are protective.

If the biofilm becomes too thick, the early colonizers get matted down and convert from aerobes, dependent on oxygen, to facultative anaerobes, which can live with or without oxygen. This basal layer forms the soil in which aggressive and opportunistic anaerobes take root. They pile up, producing a thick biofilm that crushes the architecture of the basal layer of the microfilm and closes off the oxygen channels. The dominant anaerobes produce waste products that irritate the gums.

Normally, the oral microbiome can prevent inflammation locally and at distant sites, but when the ecosystems in the mouth become imbalanced, the protective function of the microfilm is lost. As gram-positive and gram-negative bacteria colonize the surface of the tooth between teeth and at the gum line, plaque releases a number of biologically active products, including endotoxins, protein toxins, and cytokines. These irritating substances can penetrate the lining of the gums and set off an inflammatory cascade.

As the biofilm continues to grow, gum tissues produce chemical mediators, such as interleukin-1 beta (IL-1), prostaglandin, and tumor necrosis factor. These products attract white blood cells to the area and can make the blood vessels in the gums easier to penetrate, allowing proteins from blood vessels to enter the affected tissue. This is when inflammation and disease happen.

WHAT GOES WRONG IN THE MOUTH?

Healthy dental plaque is biodiverse and keeps a dynamic balance. When homeostasis is lost, the relationship of your oral microbiome with your mouth and the rest of your body can change from harmless to harmful.

It is important to note that oral diseases are among the most prevalent in the world. With the powerful mouth⇔body connection in mind, the need to keep the oral cavity healthy with a balanced microfilm is a matter of primary importance. That is why I have designed the Curatola Care Program.

TOOTH DECAY

At the macro level, the simple carbohydrates you consume—most notably sugar—ferment and produce acid that eats away at the enamel and causes tooth decay. If you consistently eat high levels of simple carbohydrates, acid production overwhelms the buffering capacity of your saliva, and your oral pH balance shifts from slightly alkaline to acidic.

When the environment favors acid-tolerant bacteria, a shift in the composition of the microbial community is likely to occur. The oral biofilm can become dominated by acid-forming and acid-tolerant bacteria, such as *mutans streptococci* and *lactobacilli*, which contribute to the acidic environment in which the bad guys can thrive and produce more plaque.

Some bacteria, seeking homeostasis, are capable of countering the production of acid from dietary sugars and can make your mouth more alkaline. But the acid lovers win sometimes, which results in tooth decay. If left untreated, the decay can penetrate into the pulp of the tooth, which becomes infected by anaerobic bacteria and dies. When the infection is located within the tooth, inflammation can easily spread to the rest of the body.

GINGIVITIS

Gingivitis, inflamed gums, is the most common bacterial disease and the mildest form of periodontal disease. It is caused by a shift in the composition of the microbial community. When anaerobic bacteria take over, which can happen when the biofilm gets too thick, they can irritate the gums. The predominant anaerobic organisms in plaque are gram-negatives, such as *Fusobacterium nucleatum*, the troublemaker discussed in Chapter 3.

If dental plaque is allowed to build too long, it becomes the hard tartar that is scraped off your teeth when they are cleaned by a dental hygienist. The thick plaque biofilm releases a number of biologically active products, including endotoxins, cytokines, and toxins. These products penetrate the outer lining of the gums, which starts a neutrophil attack and an inflammatory response that is the start of gingivitis. Bacteria in an unbalanced microbiome secrete radical or ionic oxygen in order to poke holes in cell membranes and get the cytoplasm to leak out. For anaerobes, the cytoplasm is like candy. When this happens, we see gingivitis. The condition causes changes in the color of the gums from pink to red, swelling, and bleeding.

When gingivitis is left untreated, the condition advances to periodontitis in some people. In this state, inflammation can break down gum tissue and create pockets between teeth.

When to See a Dentist

You may not even know you have gum disease or may ignore the symptoms. If you experience any symptoms from the list below, make an appointment to see your dentist or periodontist or find one if you do not get your teeth cleaned and checked regularly. Only a medical professional can evaluate how far oral disease has progressed.

The symptoms of gum disease you should look out for are:

- Bleeding gums during and after brushing
- Tender, swollen, or red gums
- Bad breath or a bad taste in the mouth that persists
- Painful chewing
- Receding gums

- Deep pockets between teeth and gums—the depth of the pocket indicates the severity of the disease.
- Loose or shifting teeth
- Changes in the way teeth fit together when you bite down

You know how gum disease can affect the rest of your body. See a dentist as soon as you notice one of these symptoms to protect your overall health.

Illustration 5: A shift from health to disease in the oral microbiome

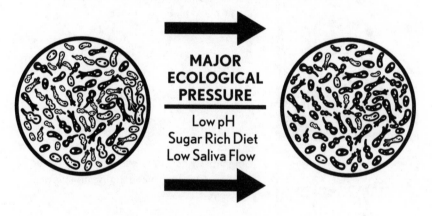

MAJOR
ECOLOGICAL
PRESSURE

Low pH
Sugar Rich Diet
Low Saliva Flow

Some pathogens (gray) may be present in low numbers in plaque or transmitted to plaque, but do not necessarily affect health in a negative way. Ecological stress is necessary for the pathogens to outcompete the residents of the microcolony (white). Ecological pressures that can lead to this shift include a diet rich in sugar, an acidic environment or low pH in the mouth, or reduced saliva flow. Aside from targeting the pathogen with antimicrobial agents that will wipe out the beneficial microbes along with the potentially harmful, it is possible to retain balance by cutting off the cause of the stress. My program is designed to help you manage the conditions that lead to disease.

PERIODONTITIS

With more severe oral disease, the inner layer of the gum and bone pull away from the teeth and form pockets. Anaerobic bacteria move right in. The body's immune system fights the bacteria by initiating an inflammatory response as the plaque spreads and grows below the gum line. If inflammation progresses, more mediators are produced that activate acute inflammation. Toxins produced by the

Illustration 6: Stages of gum disease

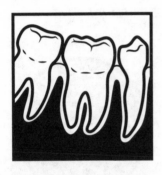

Healthy gums fit snugly around the teeth. They are firm and pink.

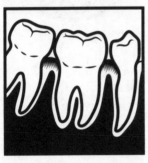

Gingivitis: Mildly inflamed gums may be red or swollen. They may bleed during brushing.

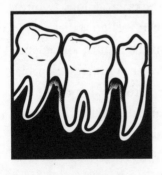

Periodontitis: Gums begin to separate and recede from the teeth, forming pockets. This allows plaque to grow toward the roots, supporting fibers, and bone.

plaque's anaerobic bacteria along with the inflammatory response start to break down the bone and connective tissue that hold teeth in place.

As the disease progresses, the pockets deepen and more gum tissue and bone are destroyed until teeth are no longer anchored in place. They become loose, and if the condition is not corrected, tooth loss occurs. Meanwhile, the markers and by-products of inflammation have easy access to the rest of the body. Since gum disease is usually not painful, it can remain untreated for years. As you already know, chronic low-grade gum disease may be more concerning for systemic health than acute gum disease.

ORAL CANCER

The sixth most prevalent cancer, oral cancer affects more than 300,000 people globally each year. As you have already read, researchers have found a correlation between the structure and function of the oral microbiome and oral cancer. As background, about 15 to 20 percent of human tumors contain pathogens derived from inflammatory infections.

The two most important risk factors for oral cancer are tobacco and alcohol. Certain strains of oral microorganisms increase the concentrations of acetaldehyde, a carcinogen, in saliva when they attempt to process alcohol and tobacco smoke.

A GRAPHIC LOOK AT THE ROOTS OF ORAL DISEASE

I like to use Illustration 7 in my keynote speeches at conferences. The graphic lays out the conditions and causes of oral problems. A balanced microbiome is dead center.

The dotted circles at the center of the grid indicate host resistance, which measures how strongly a healthy oral microbiome resists disturbance. The Curatola Care Program is designed to

Illustration 7: Acidity and inflammation

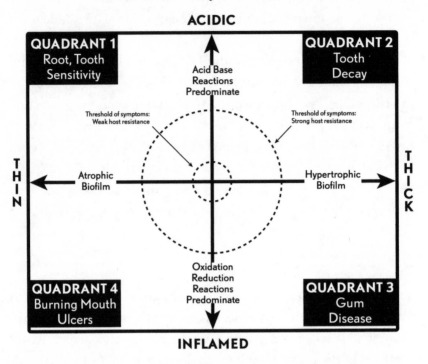

build host resistance by eliminating detergent-based, antimicrobial oral care products and establishing proper diet and nutrition, exercise, and stress management.

Chapter Five

The Ecological Catastrophe in Your Mouth

What you are about to read in this chapter is probably new to you. You might even resist what I have to say. Millions of dollars have been spent on marketing oral care products to convince you that the bacteria in your mouth have to be destroyed. Plaque is viewed as the enemy, when nothing could be further from the truth. As you have learned in the previous chapter, if the oral microcolonies are in good functioning order, plaque nourishes and protects your teeth. When balance is lost, biofilms grow too thick and harmful bacteria take over.

An unbalanced or unhealthy oral microbiome is like a garden overgrown with weeds. To get rid of the weeds, you could bulldoze the garden down to the soil. If you have any experience gardening, you know that where there is bare soil, weeds are the first plants to take root and spread. The past approach to oral care attempted to strip away the oral microbiome using detergents and emulsifiers normally found in conventional toothpastes. **More virulent microorganisms, rather than the helpful bacteria that take more time to develop, recolonize stripped-away surfaces in the mouth quickly.**

Adding to the problem, emerging science has discovered that the virulent microbes in the newly formed microfilm are often the same "friendly" organisms that were cooperative in a balanced state. **When homeostasis is disrupted, some of the beneficial microbes transform themselves into a pathogenic state.** That process is called pleomorphism, the ability of bacteria to alter their shape or size in response to adverse environmental conditions.

To continue the metaphor, **a second approach to a garden of weeds is to use herbicides. Powerful weed killers do not distinguish between weeds and desired plants— they kill everything.** That is what we have been doing since the 1970s as toothpaste and mouthwash became antimicrobial. They might "kill germs on contact," but I believe that may be harmful. The scorched earth policy results in the destruction of beneficial microbes that protect and heal teeth, gums, and mucous membranes. A balanced oral microbiome can block colonization by pathogens, a defense mechanism called colonization resistance. When you wipe out oral microcolonies with antimicrobial toothpastes and mouthwashes, you neutralize this defense.

Think of what can happen when you take a strong antibiotic that indiscriminately kills the bacteria in your gut and urogenital tracts. Disrupting stable ecosystems with antibiotics can lead to GI discomfort and bladder and genital infections. Similarly, the use of antimicrobials can promote inflammation in your mouth, which can go on to affect the rest of your body.

The oral microbiome paid a high evolutionary price to be here. Those microbes have been around longer than you have, and they exist for your benefit. You cause an ecological catastrophe every time you brush your teeth with most of today's toothpaste. This approach to oral care is overkill. Current oral hygiene is designed to be toxic to the millions of microbes that live in your mouth. **I believe it's time for doctors to get out of the pesticide business.**

A Brief History of Toothpaste

3000 to 5000 BC
Egyptians made a dental cream by mixing powdered ashes of
    oxen hooves with myrrh, burnt eggshells, pumice, and water.
    They chewed sticks to apply the dental cream.
1000 BC
Persians added burnt shells of snails and oysters along with
    gypsum, which only the rich were allowed to use.
AD 1
Ancient Romans used powdered mouse brains as toothpaste.
1780
People scrubbed their teeth with a powder that was made of
    burnt bread.
1824
A dentist named Peabody added soap to toothpaste for added
    cleanliness.
1892
Dr. Washington Sheffield was the first person to put toothpaste
    in a collapsible tube.
1914
Fluoride was added to toothpaste.
1987
"Edible" toothpaste was invented. NASA created it so that astronauts
    could brush their teeth without spitting into zero gravity.

A Brief History of Mouthwash

3000 to 5000 BC
Egyptians used many products to freshen their breath. Recipes
    have survived for chewable tablets made of dried myrrh,
    mastic, cypress grass, and lily, which were finely ground, mixed
    with honey, heated, and dried in balls.
AD 1
The Romans bought bottled Portuguese urine to purge bacteria
    from the mouth. They believed the presence of ammonia

in urine aided in disinfection and could whiten teeth. Urine remained an ingredient in mouthwash until the eighteenth century.

AD 23

People swished tortoise blood around in their mouths at least three times a year to prevent toothaches. Goat's milk was used to maintain good breath, and white wine was used as a rinse.

AD 40 to 90

Dioscorides, a Greek surgeon and physician, recommended that a mixture of the juice and leaves of olives, gum, myrrh, pomegranate, vinegar, and wine could help to fight bad breath.

Twelfth Century

St. Hildegard von Bingen, a German mystic, suggested that swishing pure, cold water around in the mouth could help remove tartar.

Sixteenth Century

Mint and vinegar rinsing solutions were believed to rid the mouth of bad breath and germs during the Middle Ages.

Nineteenth Century

Mouthwashes as we know them today developed in the late 1800s. Alcohol was added to help fight germs and bacteria. One of the most popular mouthwashes today, Listerine, was invented as an antiseptic to clean operating rooms and began to be used to bathe wounds.

1914

Listerine was introduced as a mouthwash that killed germs.

TIME TO REPLACE TODAY'S ORAL CARE

Invented by soap makers more than one hundred years ago, toothpaste as we know it is flavored detergent used in the mouth to scrub the surfaces clean of bacteria. With the addition of antimicrobial agents, toothpaste wipes out the oral microbiome by sterilizing your mouth. The common approach to managing the oral microbiome today is to strip it down to the pellicle with detergents in combination with antimicrobial agents to slow or prevent recolonization.

The alcohol in mouthwash disturbs, denatures, and dehydrates your oral ecosystem. Both toothpaste and mouthwash clear the way for pathogens to proliferate, because they kill off the microbes that exist to keep opportunistic invaders in check. **Oral hygiene today turns on a pathogenic switch.** Everyday oral care is more than ineffective; it is harmful. Despite the use of antimicrobial oral products, the number of adults with gum disease has not changed forty years later. Though tooth decay is down, gum disease has stayed at just about the same level. You would expect a better outcome if the scorched earth policy actually worked.

Even more alarming, I believe there is an historical connection between sterilizing the mouth, which came into practice in the 1970s, and the catastrophic rise we have witnessed in diseases such as obesity, diabetes, cardiovascular disease, and metabolic syndrome. Of course, many factors are responsible for the epidemic proportions these illnesses have reached, but rendering the oral microbiome ineffective in its protective role and creating a climate in the mouth in which pathogens thrive certainly contribute to the health crisis today. You have read about the effects of the mouth⇔body connection. The epidemic rise of many diseases today parallels the use of antimicrobials in oral care.

Since the antimicrobial concept of oral care took hold, many studies have found that sterilizing the mouth has improved oral health, but no one was aware of the importance of the oral microbiome in overall health when these studies were done. New research is examining what we may be sacrificing by wiping out the microbial communities in the mouth. **Overzealous oral hygiene is being recognized as a cause of disease.**

An aspect of cardiovascular disease, the No. 1 killer in the United States for men and women, illustrates this dynamic. The oral microbiome has a role in nitrate metabolism, which affects cardiovascular health. About a quarter of the nitrate you consume in food is returned to your mouth in saliva. Facultative anaerobes in the tongue biofilm reduce nitrate to nitrite, which is then swallowed. Some of the nitrite is converted in the stomach to nitrous oxide. Essential for vascular health, nitrous oxide helps to keep blood vessels pliant and supple, which prevents high blood pressure. The central role of oral bacteria in this process has been confirmed. **Studies have found that the increase in nitrite in the bloodstream after eating foods that contain nitrate is markedly reduced when antimicrobial mouth rinse is used.** This natural mechanism for maintaining cardiovascular health appears to stop working efficiently when the oral microbiome is thrown off-balance by antimicrobial mouth rinse.

THE NEW GOAL

Rather than stripping the microfilm from your mouth, my goal is to drive the ecosystem to its low-film thickness and an odorless, protective, slick, and slippery state. I have been working on a way to make it difficult for the high-film thickness microfilm to maintain itself without killing it off with detergents, antimicrobials, or alcohol. I have spent the past ten years developing a toothpaste I call Revitin®, which supports a healthy oral microbiome.

As you have learned, a thick ecosystem has needs that are very different from a balanced one. We have to exploit the difference. The Curatola Care Program offers ways to control the composition of plaque by regulating natural homeostasis to maintain normal metabolic activity of oral biofilms. **To return to the garden image, my aim is to use the principles of organic gardening to support the microorganisms and biochemistry that favor a healthy microbiome.** I have found that this goal can be achieved quickly, because the speed of maturation and biochemical turnover are much faster on the level of microorganisms.

In Part 1, you have gained an understanding of the powerful mouth⇔body connection and the importance of this two-way street to your overall health. In Part 2, I shift focus from a scientific look at the mouth's effect on the body to what you have to do to protect your oral microbiome and to reduce devastating inflammation in your body. You will start by learning how to clean up your act and detoxify, and then move on to how to eat for balance in your mouth and body. Exercise follows. Working out at high intensity just two times a week for fifteen minutes is all that is required for big benefits. Of course, moving more is essential, but I consider that recreation. If your goal is to reduce inflammation, stress relief has to be a major part of the program. Part 2 gives you the fundamentals for a plan of action, guidelines for a way to live that will boost the health of your mouth and your body.

PART II

THE FUNDAMENTALS

Chapter Six

Climate Control

Time to Clean Up

Research spurred by World War II launched a chemical age that profoundly changed the world and improved our lives immeasurably. On the down side, there is a price to pay for convenience. Every day, whether you know it or not, you are walking through an environment that is a toxic minefield. From the couch you are sitting on to your shampoo to your easy-care clothing, you can be exposing yourself to toxins, which can build up in your cells and organs over time.

Your body was not designed to deal with the thousands of manmade chemicals that are poisoning you from the air you breathe, the water you drink, the food you eat, the cleaning and grooming products you use, and even the clothes you wear. The unprecedented high level of toxins in the environment can overwhelm your body's ability to process and eliminate these poisons. When toxins accumulate in your body, they interrupt your metabolic functions. Your immune system goes into overdrive in an attempt to expel the foreign substances. As a result, your body becomes inflamed and acidic.

Americans on average use forty pounds of toxic cleaning products a year. Eighty percent of the chemicals found in everyday products lack detailed information about their toxicity. The chemicals found in your cleaning products, your clothing, your grooming products, and your home are absorbed through your skin and your breath. These toxins make their way into the environment when they are poured down the drain, sprayed into the air, tossed into the trash, or flushed down the toilet.

The average American woman uses 515 chemical ingredients on her body every day. More than fifteen thousand ingredients are approved for use in grooming products in the United States, but 90 percent of those ingredients have never been tested for health effects. Though the European Union has banned the use of 1,100 ingredients in cosmetics, the Food and Drug Administration in this country has prohibited only ten ingredients for cosmetic use.

There is little you can do to protect yourself from some environmental toxins, but you can make informed choices about the food you eat, the cleaning and grooming products you use, and the clothing you wear. **My rule of thumb is to select products that are as close to nature as possible.** Read labels carefully. If you cannot pronounce an ingredient, you probably should avoid it.

Toxins are everywhere, and you may be exposed from unexpected sources. For example:

- Cell phones, computers, televisions, and microwaves outgas or emit fumes of BPAs and other toxic chemicals as well as disrupt electromagnetic fields.
- Most carpets, upholstered furniture, and pressed or treated wood outgas formaldehyde and other toxins.
- Synthetic fabrics are petroleum based and processed with many chemicals.
- Wrinkle-resistant, stain-resistant, and drip-dry fabrics all have toxic finishes.
- Scratched nonstick pots and pans can be deadly.
- Mattresses contain flame-retardants by law. Those chemicals are neurotoxins.
- Polyurethane finishes outgas toxic fumes.

- Vinyl flooring is toxic.
- Conventional dry cleaning residues are powerful neuro-toxins.
- Most food cans are lined with plastic that leaches into the contents.
- Plastic food containers and wraps, unless marked BPA free, along with food packaging contain highly toxic substances.
- Even plastic toys can be toxic unless they are labeled BPA free.

Toxin Patrol at Home

Keep your eyes open when you read the labels on the products you use.

Watch out for these chemicals:

1. **Arsenic** is found in drinking water and treated lumber.

2. **Bisphenol A (BPA)** is one of the most common chemicals in the world, but it is being controlled. Some plastic bottles, the lining of metal food cans, reusable food containers, electronic equipment, and even many tooth-colored dental fillings called composite all contain BPA. Every time you send an e-mail, make a call on your cell phone, put on your sunglasses, or run your tongue over a composite filling in your tooth—more about this soon—you may be in contact with this endocrine disruptor.

3. **Chlorine bleach** is an ingredient in many household cleaners. Chlorine is a highly toxic gas. It is considered a pesticide under the Federal Hazardous Substances Act.

4. **Formaldehyde** serves as a disinfectant, a preservative, and a glue in pressed wood products. You will find it in most furniture, carpets, dishwashing liquids, fabric softeners, carpet cleaners, and permanent press fabrics.

5. **Perfluorinated chemicals (PFCs)** are used to make stain repellants, nonstick surfaces on pots and pans, and microwave popcorn bags.

6. **Phthalates** soften plastics, such as toys, shower curtains, plastic bags, and food wraps. They give lotions their texture.

7. **Polybrominated diethyl ethers (PBDEs)** are flame-retardants found in televisions, computers, mattresses, and furniture.

8. **Polyvinyl chloride** is a plastic used in most flooring, window frames, and pipes.

9. **Triclosan** is an antibacterial found in most conventional toothpastes, dish detergents, liquid hand soaps, and bedding. Since Triclosan is an ingredient in most toothpastes, I will discuss this toxin at length later in this chapter. In September 2016, the Food and Drug Administration banned the use of triclosan in antimicrobial hand soap, but this dangerous hormone disruptor is still allowed to be an ingredient in toothpaste. Go figure.

10. **Volatile organic compounds (VOCs)** are gases and vapors that contain carbons, which contribute to air pollution. VOCs outgas from conventional cleaning and personal grooming products, carpets, paints, air fresheners, and dry cleaning.

The world today is a toxic place, and most of the toxins to which you are exposed inflame your body. Since your mouth is a gateway at the front line of defense, a healthy environment in your mouth can protect your body from toxic invaders that can leach into your gums, bloodstream, and cells. A well–balanced microbiome is a strong advance guard against the toxins you encounter in everyday life. This chapter gives you a game plan for protecting the environment in your mouth with specific recommendations for change, beginning with dropping the scorched earth approach to oral care.

WHY IS THERE A POISON WARNING ON TOOTHPASTE?

In case you have not noticed, there is a warning on most commercial toothpastes that reads:

Warning
Keep out of reach of children under 6 years of age. If more than used for brushing is accidentally swallowed, get medical help or contact a Poison Control Center right away.

After setting the minimum age for toothpaste use at two, the directions go on to read:

Do not swallow.
To minimize swallowing use a pea-sized amount in children under 6.

According to the Columbia University College of Dental Medicine, the lethal dose of fluoride for an eight-year-old child weighing 45 pounds is 655 milligrams. Your child would have to consume more than four tubes of toothpaste to reach this level. For a two-year-old, 22-pound child, the lethal dose is 320 milligrams, or more than two full tubes of toothpaste. Several highly toxic substances appear on the ingredients list on most tubes of commercial toothpaste. They include:

- Sodium fluoride
- Sodium lauryl sulfate
- Triclosan
- Artificial sweeteners
- Artificial color dyes
- Propylene glycol

- Diethanolamine (DEA)
- Microbeads

I might as well start the discussion with the most controversial ingredient.

THE FLUORIDE CONTROVERSY

I could not write a chapter on toxins without weighing in on the fluoride controversy. Fluoride, which is derived from one of the single most reactive nonradioactive elements on the Periodic Table of Elements, was added to the water supply in the United States in the 1940s for the purpose of reducing cavities. The sacred cow of preventive dentistry, fluoride has been promoted as one of the top ten most important public health measures in the twentieth century.

According to the Centers for Disease Control, 90 percent of the fluoride added to public water supplies is actually not sodium fluoride at all. It is fluorosilicic acid, a waste product that comes from chemicals produced as by-products from the manufacture of phosphate fertilizers and aluminum manufacturing. Fluorosilicic acid is used in manufacturing commercial detergents such as cryolite, silicon tetrafluoride, and other fluosilicates. Its corrosive acidic nature leaches the lead and arsenic from water delivery plumbing, which is suspected happened with the toxic water in Flint, Michigan. On the other hand, sodium fluoride in toothpastes and other products is an ingredient in rat and roach poisons and industrial pesticides. Sodium fluoride also serves as a key component of anesthetic, hypnotic, and psychiatric drugs.

Under the banner of Preventive Dentistry, most Americans are really being "medicated" with industrial waste products that are already poisoning the environment. Roughly 99 percent of fluoridated water never touches our teeth. It is used for showering, watering crops, and washing clothes.

Some antifluoride activists believe that water fluoridation allows industry to profit from dumping hazardous waste, rather than paying for disposal.

Though fluoride is added to public water supplies in amounts thought to be "safe," you are now exposed to more sources of fluoride than when it was first introduced into the water supply. Toothpaste and mouthwash enhanced with fluoride, food processed with fluoridated water, and fluoride added to multivitamins have greatly increased the amount of fluoride to which you are exposed. Overexposure to fluoride has many negative effects.

In toothpaste, fluoride is supposed to bind to tooth enamel to make the tooth more resistant to acid attack from bacteria. Whether and how much fluoride protects teeth are not clear. Fluoride's role in the decline of tooth decay is now in serious doubt. One thing is known for certain: Excess fluoridation has led to fluorosis, a discoloring and weakening of enamel. This condition occurs when fluoride interferes with the cells that produce enamel, creating white flecks and stripes on the teeth.

The fact is that children are being overexposed to fluoride. Four out of ten adolescents have some level of fluorosis. **The Environmental Protection Agency listed fluoride as one of the hundred chemicals for which there is substantial evidence of developmental neurotoxicity. That's right, fluoride damages the developing brain.** Other studies have reported an association between fluoride exposure and reduced IQ. Two recent studies have linked fluoridation to ADHD and underactive thyroid. The studies have been alarming. The tide is turning against water fluoridation. Research has found insufficient evidence that fluoridation reduces tooth decay in adults. The new science of the oral microbiome has shown its ability to remineralize teeth by facilitating the transport of ionic calcium and phosphorus from saliva to the surface of tooth enamel. Keeping your oral microbiome in a healthy balance is a healthier approach to preventing decay, along with good diet and nutrition.

SEVEN MORE TOXINS YOU ARE EXPOSED TO EVERY TIME YOU BRUSH YOUR TEETH

Many name-brand toothpastes and mouthwashes contain potentially harmful ingredients that may penetrate through the tissue of your mouth, enter your bloodstream, and build up in your liver, kidneys, heart, lungs, and tissues. Just read the label on the toothpaste or mouthwash in your medicine cabinet. You'll see that, in addition to sodium fluoride, they are loaded with other dangerous toxins and chemicals, such as triclosan, sodium lauryl sulfate, artificial color, artificial sweeteners, diethanolamine (DEA), propylene glycol, and microbeads. Once you are aware of how harmful these common ingredients can be, you will be as eager as my patients are to clean up their act. Why expose yourself to toxins if you can easily avoid it? Let's take a look at these dangerous ingredients.

GOING AFTER MICROBES WITH PESTICIDE: TRICLOSAN

Triclosan is an antibacterial chemical that has been shown to prevent gum disease. **The United States Environmental Protection Agency has registered triclosan as a dangerous pesticide, a human health risk, and an environmental risk.** This type of pesticide can be stored in body fat and accumulate to toxic levels.

Triclosan is a chlorophenol, which is a class of chemicals that is suspected of causing cancer in humans. Taken internally, even in small amounts, phenol can lead to cold sweats, circulatory collapse, convulsions, coma, and death. Long-term exposure and repeated use of many pesticide products can damage the liver, kidneys, heart, and lungs; suppress the immune system; and cause hormonal disruption, paralysis, sterility, and brain hemorrhages. Triclosan has also been linked to antibiotic resistance. Knowing the harmful effects of triclosan should make you wonder why the FDA still allows its use as an ingredient in toothpaste.

Researchers at Virginia Tech have found that when triclosan is mixed with chlorine found in tap water, chloroform is formed. When inhaled or swallowed, chloroform affects the brain, liver, and kidneys. Chloroform was used as an anesthetic during surgery for many years before its harmful effects were recognized.

More than 95 percent of the triclosan in consumer products goes down the drain. Triclosan destroys ecological balance when it contaminates wastewater. Exposure to sunlight in water transforms triclosan to dioxin, a highly toxic compound that affects algae and aquatic ecosystems. According to a United States Geological Survey study of organic wastewater contaminants in streams, triclosan was one of the most frequently detected compounds found at some of the highest concentrations. You should get this toxin out of your mouth.

Triclosan is marketed under more than a dozen different names, including Microban, Irgasan, Biofresh, Lexol-300, Ster-Zac, and Cloxifenolum. Keep this in mind when you are reading labels.

BRUSHING YOUR TEETH WITH COAL TAR AND CRUDE OIL: FD&C BLUE DYES 1 AND 2

Some toothpaste companies use artificial dyes and colorings to make their products more appealing. These dyes were originally made from coal tar oil, which is a sticky, black by-product of petroleum distillation and steel manufacturing. Some of the complex chemicals isolated from coal tar were found to be active carcinogens, which led to government regulations and restrictions.

Today, coal tar dyes are synthetic, engineered rather than extracted from coal tar. Even so, the dyes continue to have carcinogenic properties, which is why they are still called coal tar dyes. **You do not have to swallow toothpaste to suffer the**

negative effects of coal tar dyes. The carcinogens can be quickly absorbed through the mucous membranes in your mouth or the skin on your lips and find their way into your blood and cells.

Recent studies indicate that FD&C Blue Dyes 1 and 2 can trigger a wide number of behavioral, learning, and health problems.

FD&C color dyes may also cause potentially severe allergic reactions, asthma attacks, headaches, nausea, fatigue, nervousness, lack of concentration, and cancer. I think you will agree that the color of your toothpaste or mouthwash should not be harmful to your health.

FOAMING AT THE MOUTH: SODIUM LAURYL SULFATE (SLS) OR SODIUM LAURETH SULFATE

Sodium lauryl sulfate and sodium laureth sulfate are emulsifiers and foaming agents that are a common ingredient in many personal care products, including some toothpastes. SLS is the active compound in some insecticides, particularly those targeting fruit flies. It is sometimes used in flea and tick shampoo for cats and dogs. This inexpensive ingredient can be found in many industrial-cleaning agents, such as engine degreasers, car wash soaps, and garage floor cleaners.

SLS, a surfactant, breaks the surface tension of water, allowing bubbles to form, and separates molecules to allow a better interaction between toothpaste and your teeth. As a result, **SLS has the power of penetration. This chemical can accumulate in the brain, heart, and liver with potentially harmful effects.** SLS is corrosive and irritating to skin tissue. This chemical can cause microscopic tears in your mouth that can lead to canker sores. SLS can mess with your taste buds, enhancing bitter tastes, which is one reason food tastes bad right after you brush your teeth.

You do not need foam to brush your teeth. SLS is put to better use at a car wash as it floats the grease away.

USING AIRPLANE DEICER TO CLEAN YOUR TEETH—PROPYLENE GLYCOL

The active ingredient in antifreeze, propylene glycol is an alcohol that acts as a wetting agent and surfactant in toothpaste. This mineral oil is also used in paints and enamels as well as airplane deicers. Prolonged contact with the chemical, even at reduced concentrations, can lead to rapid absorption through the skin, which can promote brain, liver, and kidney abnormalities. **Though the EPA (Environmental Protection Agency) prohibits workers from handling propylene glycol without wearing rubber gloves, the chemical is still used in common health care products like some conventional toothpaste.** Isn't that enough to persuade you not to put this ingredient in your mouth?

It appears on labels under different names: 1,2 dihycroxypropane, 1,2-propanediol, 2-hydroxypropanol, methylethyl glycol, propane-1,2-diol, 1,2-dihydroxypropane, 1,2-proplylene glycol, alpha-propyleneglycol, Dowfrost, and methylethylene glycol.

HIGH ON THE TOXICITY SCALE: DIETHANOLAMINE (DEA)

DEA, another foaming product used in some conventional toothpaste, has been ranked 10—as toxic as it gets—by the Environmental Working Group (www.EWG.org). DEA can disrupt hormones and forms cancer-causing nitrates. **The EWG has linked DEA with stomach cancer, bladder cancer, liver cancer, and organ system toxicity.** Ask yourself this: Is having your toothpaste foam worth the risk of developing cancer?

Julia, a cancer patient on a chemotherapy regimen, came to see me because she was suffering from painful sores in her mouth and on her tongue. She assumed it was a reaction to all the strong chemicals she was being exposed to.

I gave her a tube of Revitin, the toothpaste I developed. Within a week, her mouth was looking better, and the pain was reduced. In a month's time, the sores were completely gone. Whether the condition of her mouth was a reaction to her medication, her immune system was out of whack, or her mouth was ultrasensitive to the toxins in the toothpaste she was using, once her oral microbiome was back in balance, the problem in her mouth resolved.

HOW SWEET IT'S NOT: ARTIFICIAL SWEETENERS

Saccharin, aspartame, xylitol, and erythritol are commonly used to mask the bitter chemical taste of toothpaste. Manufactured from petroleum products, saccharin and aspartame are approximately 350 times sweeter than sugar. Saccharin can cause bladder cancer and has been tied to weight gain. The Food and Drug Administration advised that it be banned, but their recommendation was not put into effect.

The body breaks down aspartame into the toxic by-products formic acid and formaldehyde, a potent neurotoxin and a carcinogen. Aspartame has been linked to migraines, memory loss, seizures, Parkinson's disease, and brain tumors.

Some toothpastes contain xylitol and erythritol, known as sugar alcohols. Xylitol has become the "darling of sugar substitutes," the margarine of the artificial sweetener industry. **Though touted as a "natural" sweetener, sugar alcohols are produced by hydrogenating sugar with the use of a heavy metal catalyst called Raney nickel, a powdered nickel-aluminum alloy.** Hydrogenation is the same process used to make margarines and other pro-inflammatory foods. Though xylitol can be derived from the xylan of birch trees, using xylan from corncobs is much less expensive. Of course, genetically modified (GMO) corn is used.

Sugar alcohols are metabolic disruptors. Xylitol, an antiplaque agent, contributes to gut and oral microbiome imbalance. It is not broken down in the stomach and is poorly absorbed, which can lead to fermentation causing intestinal gas, cramps, and diarrhea.

Using the same industrial process as xylitol, erythritol, found in Truvia, is derived mostly from GMO corn. Researchers claim that erythritol can be used as an insecticide against fruit flies. Truvia-fed fruit flies had difficulty climbing up a small vial, because their motor function was impaired. This did not occur with six other sweeteners tested.

Unlike xylitol, erythritol is well absorbed in the gut, but poorly metabolized. Erythritol contributes to acidosis, which can lead to acid reflux and an increased risk of cancer in the larynx. This artificial sweetener may promote dehydration, creating feelings of excessive thirst.

The effects of artificial sweeteners cover a broad range of "feeling off" symptoms: headaches, dizziness, mood changes, nausea, memory loss, joint pain, depression, anxiety, and blurred vision. If you want to enhance your sense of well-being, it makes sense to avoid artificial sweeteners wherever you encounter them.

EXFOLIATORS THAT DON'T GO AWAY: POLYETHYLENE MICROBEADS

Tiny plastic particles, the same plastic from which kitchen trash bags are made, are used in many facial and body scrubs as exfoliators and in many toothpastes for color and texture. The problem is that the tiny pellets are not biodegradable and are too small to be caught in water treatment plants. They end up in waterways, where they act as sponges, absorbing pesticides, phthalates, and heavy metals. Fish can mistake them for food, and the toxins they consume move up the food chain.

When used in toothpaste, the microbeads can get stuck between the teeth and under the gums, where they can trap bacteria that lead to gingivitis. You don't want your toothpaste to promote gum disease.

Fortunately, the Microbead-Free Waters Act of 2015 requires companies to stop using plastic microbeads by June 2017. They may be replaced by biodegradable substitutes. You don't want these in your toothpaste either.

DON'T BE FOOLED BY "NATURAL" TOOTHPASTES

It is easy to confuse "natural" with "nontoxic." Though many "natural" toothpastes have removed fluoride, they can replace the chemical with fluorspar, a natural mineral. When this mineral is processed, it can find its way into natural toothpaste to "prevent cavities." Fluorspar is used mainly in the chemical industry to manufacture hydrofluoric acid (HF), which is then used to manufacture a variety of products including highly toxic fluorocarbon chemicals, foam blowing agents, refrigerants, and a variety of fluoride chemicals. It is an ingredient in steel and iron, cement and ceramics, nuclear fuel, and Teflon. **Do not be tricked into thinking that fluorspar is a healthy substitute for sodium fluoride.**

Sodium bicarbonate, often used as a whitening agent in many natural toothpastes, is abrasive and damaging to tooth enamel. Tooth enamel remineralizes daily from the supply of ionic calcium and phosphorus in the saliva. **Scratching the surface of the tooth with an abrasive such as sodium bicarbonate can harm the enamel and prevent remineralization. Its action on the tooth is much like sandblasting.** In fact, sodium bicarbonate is used in many commercial blasting applications for paint removal.

Sodium lauryl sulfate is often used as an ingredient in "natural" toothpaste as well. Though SLS can be made from natural ingredients such as coconut oil or palm kernel oil, it can still act as an irritant.

You will find xylitol or erythritol in most so-called natural toothpastes. Remember, xylitol is an antimicrobial sugar alcohol mostly derived from GMO corn and synthesized by a hydrogenation process, which uses a heavy metal in its manufacture. That combination of factors is all you need to know to say no to sugar alcohols.

As you have read in the previous pages, you want to avoid the scorched earth policy to your oral microbiome. Herbal antimicrobials in toothpaste such as peppermint, cinnamon, and licorice can have the same antimicrobial effect as synthetic chemicals. For example, tea tree oil, derived from an Australian evergreen, is a powerful antimicrobial. It can be toxic to pets and can cause toxic and allergic reactions in humans, especially if swallowed. Serious side effects include confusion, inability to walk, rash, and hormonal imbalances. Tea tree oil, like many other natural substances, can be poisonous if used in the wrong way, in the case of toothpaste that means swallowed. In 2008, poison centers in the United States received more than twice as many calls about tea tree oil than any other named essential oil. Licorice root and tulsi oil, made from the Indian holy basil plant, are also used for their powerful antimicrobial properties in "natural" toothpaste, which can cause havoc in your mouth's ecosystems.

The daughter of one of my patients was sensitive to every toothpaste, which produced painful sores in her mouth. She began using Revitin, the toothpaste I developed to restore a balanced oral microbiome, and her mouth healed immediately.

The drugs to treat cancer can cause many oral problems. Revitin has healed the mouths of many of my patients with cancer.

BRUSHING YOUR TEETH SHOULD BE ORAL THERAPY

I worked with my New York University College of Dentistry classmate and business partner, Dr. David Shuch, for more than fifteen years to develop a naturopathic toothpaste, which we called Revitin®. Recognizing the "revitalizing and vitamin-rich" formulation, we decided on that name. Revitin was designed to restore balance to the oral microbiome instead of stripping the mouth's ecosystem as conventional toothpastes do. When I see there is room for improvement in my field, I do something about it.

Revitin is all-natural, toxin free, detergent free, and antibacterial free. There is no poison warning on the tube. Revitin does not contain any harmful chemicals or additives I have mentioned, including artificial colors or sweeteners, peroxide, triclosan, or sodium laurel sulfate.

The core of Revitin's proprietary formulation are called NuPath Bioactives, a blend of key antioxidants, prebiotic micronutrients, herbal extracts, and microminerals to support a balanced ecosystem in the mouth. The ingredients include:

Coenzyme Q10, Vitamin C, Vitamin E, MSM, cranberry seed extract, xanthan gum, quillaja extract, calcium carbonate, vegetable glycerin, hydrated silica, stevia, and natural essential oils for flavor.

The ingredients in Revitin are prebiotic, homeopathic, and naturopathic. Prebiotics are now considered possibly more effective in nourishing and supporting our microbial communities than probiotics. In the gut, these prebiotic ingredients include fibers such as inulin. In the mouth, probiotics have been shown to be ineffective due to the protective nature of the indigenous oral microbes that make the environment very inhospitable to "pro" or "con" -biotics.

On the other hand, prebiotics in the mouth such as xanthan gum and cranberry seed oil, along with prebiotic-like vitamins and nutrients, create a very healthy and robust oral microbiome. Revitin acts like a smart toothpaste by respecting and working with the natural ecology of the mouth, instead of stripping away healthy bacteria as many commercial brands do.

In other words, it does not rely on natural or synthetic anti-microbial or antibiotic agents. Aside from working with your mouth's natural defenses, Revitin conditions your gums. Our goal was to create a toothpaste that would help smokers, reduce sensitivity, comfort ulcers, heal trauma, stop gum bleeding, and thin plaque buildup.

You are about to witness a revolution in oral care because of all the new findings about the oral microbiome and the mouth⇔body connection. It is time to abandon an approach that is almost a half century old and replace it with alternatives that protect the integrity of your oral microbiome.

Recommended Toothpastes

My top recommendation is the "oral microbiome supportive toothpaste I developed, Revitin Prebiotic Toothpaste. It is all-natural and works with the natural defenses of the oral microbiome. Several studies have been done to confirm its effectiveness, and I believe Revitin is the best on the market. It is available online at http://revitin.com/prebiotic-toothpaste/.

If you want to try other toothpastes in the natural category, I recommend:

- Revitin Prebiotic Toothpaste Citrus Clean Flavor, $12, www.revitin.com
- Auromere Ayurvedic Licorice Toothpaste, $6, www.auromere.com
- Weleda Calendula Toothpaste, $8, www.usa.weleda.com
- Hello Natural Sweet Mint, $5, www.target.com

- Honest Natural and Fluoride Free Toothpaste, $6, www.honest
  .com
- David's Premium Natural Toothpaste, $8, www.davids-usa.com
- Botanique Himalaya Original Neem and Pomegranate
  Toothpaste, $6, www.Himalayausa.com
- Dr. Bronner's All-One Anise or Cinnamon Toothpaste, $6.49,
  www.drbronner.com
  (All prices are subject to change.)

Replacing the commercial toothpaste you are using with one that will support the health of your mouth is an easy thing to do. The benefits far outweigh the energy you expend to make the change.

MAKE YOUR OWN TOOTHPASTE AND MOUTHWASH

If you want to avoid toothpaste and mouthwashes with carcinogenic chemicals and other harmful ingredients found in conventional toothpaste, there is no reason you cannot make your own oral care products. Though there are products available that pass my safety test (see list on pages 85–86), you might want to give it a try. If you cannot find the ingredients in your local health food store or Whole Foods, these items are readily available online.

Homemade toothpaste allows you to control what is in it. You will not have to worry about the warning sign not to swallow the toothpaste that you find on most tubes of commercial toothpaste, because you can leave out the toxins. At the same time, you can select the flavor and the level of sweetness that appeals to you. Not only will you save money, but making your own toothpaste will also help the environment by reducing the amount of packaging that ends up in landfills.

Homemade Toothpaste

This is a recipe I developed for this book:

- 4 teaspoons calcium carbonate powder (for whitening and remineralizing)
- 2 teaspoons xanthan gum (for binding and a good source of prebiotic fiber)
- 1 teaspoon organic vegetable glycerin (for binding and providing a smooth consistency)
- 10 drops organic liquid stevia (sweet but not too sweet)
- 1/8 teaspoon Himalayan salt (anti-inflammatory, remineralizing, and a source of trace minerals)
- 10 drops sea buckthorn oil (loaded with omegas and Vitamins C and E and great for gums)
- 10 drops spearmint or cinnamon essential oil or 5 drops lemon or other citrus essential oil (for breath freshening and flavor)
- ¼ cup filtered water

In a large glass mixing cup, stir together the calcium powder, silica, xanthan gum, glycerin, and liquid stevia.

Add the Himalayan salt, sea buckthorn oil, and essential oil.

Add the water slowly and mix to the consistency of sour cream. The paste will thicken over time.

Pour or scrape the mixture into a glass jar or bottle with a tight screw cap.

Close the lid and stir ingredients occasionally to maintain consistency.

The toothpaste can stay in the jar in the bathroom.

Homemade Mouthwash

While you are making your toothpaste, you may want to try your hand at mouthwash that will not exterminate the microbial life in your mouth. You also want to avoid alcohol, which is harsh and drying. Here is a recipe I like for mouthwash that whitens and remineralizes:

- 2 teaspoons calcium carbonate powder (for whitening and remineralizing)
- 10 drops organic liquid stevia (sweet but not too sweet)

1/8 teaspoon Himalayan salt (anti-inflammatory, remineralizing, and a source of trace minerals)

10 drops sea buckthorn oil (loaded with omegas and Vitamins C and E and great for gums)

10 drops spearmint or cinnamon essential oil (for breath freshening and flavor)

2 cups filtered water

In a large glass mixing cup, stir together the calcium powder and liquid stevia.

Add the Himalayan salt, sea buckthorn oil, and essential oil.

Add the water and stir.

Pour the mixture into a glass jar or bottle with a tight screw cap.

Close the lid and shake the ingredients together for about 30 to 60 seconds, until the salt and calcium carbonate powder dissolves.

Shake well before using as oils can separate.

Use as needed 1 to 2 times a day for 30 to 60 seconds.

The mouthwash can stay in the jar in the bathroom. Refrigerating the mouthwash would make the oils separate more.

---

10 Ways to Keep the Dazzle in Your Smile

Everyone knows the basics—brush twice a day and floss at least once—but the following practical tips will keep your mouth healthy and boost the wattage of your smile:

1. **Don't be hard on your teeth.** Use a soft toothbrush, not medium or hard. Soft nylon bristles with rounded ends will not hurt your gums. Hard brushes are too abrasive. They can make your gums bleed and wear down your teeth. An aggressive brushing technique can damage your gums. Brush your teeth gently at a 45-degree angle, in a circular motion. Ten to twenty percent of the adult population has tooth and gum damage due to overbrushing.

2. **Brush with the radio on.** You should brush your teeth three to four minutes, the average length of a song. People tend to brush one minute twice a day, which is not enough time to do a thorough job. Try dancing while you're at it.

3. **Try an electric toothbrush if you need motivation to brush longer.** Electric toothbrushes don't work that much better than manual ones, but they do cover more area faster and provide a distraction. The tufts of nylon bristles, which move in a rotary motion, can cause your gums to bleed at first. Use light force and slow movements to protect your gums. The action of an electric or battery-operated toothbrush can reduce gingivitis.

4. **Air-dry your equipment.** After a good rinse with water when you have finished brushing, store your toothbrush in an upright position and allow it to dry before using it again. Avoid covering toothbrushes or storing them in closed containers, which can promote the growth of bacteria. When using a storage container, be certain to use one that allows air to circulate so that your toothbrush can breathe. If you keep a toothbrush at the office, let it dry before putting it in a container. Change a work toothbrush often, because bacteria can build up when it is stored in a desk drawer.

5. **A toothbrush is not forever.** Old toothbrushes with frayed bristles are not only ineffective but can harbor bacteria that cause inflammation. Change your toothbrush or replace the head of your electric toothbrush every three to four months or sooner if the bristles show signs of wear.

6. **Number 1 in gum disease prevention—flossing every day.** Nothing works better to prevent gum inflammation than flossing for two to three minutes at least once a day. Flossing removes bacteria left behind from food particles that get stuck between teeth. If you avoid flossing because it irritates your gums, be patient. Your gums will toughen up the more you floss. Do you find flossing hard to handle?

You can choose from a number of interdental cleaners, such as wooden or plastic sticks or brushes designed to clean between the teeth. Forget about toothpicks, because they can injure your gums. An oral irrigator, which shoots a stream of water, might work to dislodge food particles from between your teeth. Flossing before brushing can make it easier for the bristles of the toothbrush to get between your teeth.

7. **Don't brush too soon after eating.** When you eat or drink acidic foods and beverages, such as sugary energy and carbonated drinks, wine, coffee, and tomatoes, wait at least thirty minutes to an hour before brushing. If you don't, you are just brushing acid into the enamel. Rinse your mouth out with water if you feel the need to clean your teeth soon after eating.

8. **Chew sugarless gum after meals and snacks.** Gum increases your saliva production, prevents cavity-causing bacteria from attaching to your teeth, and can dislodge particles stuck between your teeth.

9. **Use a straw to drink decay-promoting sugary beverages or coffee and tea, which can stain.** Doing this will minimize the amount of time the sugar or staining liquids are in contact with your teeth.

10. **Only use a mouthwash without alcohol.** Aside from killing off good and bad bacteria, alcohol can dry out the moist tissues in your mouth and cause ulcers. Recent studies have shown a correlation between using mouthwashes more than three times a day and increased oral cancer risk.

MEDICATIONS CAN SUBVERT ORAL BALANCE

Certain medications can affect the state of your mouth. That is why I ask my patients to give me a full list of the medications they are taking, including prescriptions, over-the-counter medications, vitamins, and supplements. Medicines to treat depression, allergies, high blood pressure, cancer, and even a cold can have a bad effect on your oral health.

> Warning: Do not stop taking a medication if you think it is having an oral side effect. If you are having oral problems and are taking a medication you find listed in this section, discuss your concern with your doctor, who can suggest ways to correct the problem. Your health care provider may be able to prescribe an alternative medication that will not have the same effect.

The best way to discuss this material is to organize medications according to common side effects.

DRY MOUTH

More than four hundred medicines are associated with dry mouth, a significant problem. If your cleansing and remineralizing saliva is not flowing normally, the tissues in your mouth can become irritated and inflamed. You will be more likely to develop gum disease and tooth decay. Some of the medications that list dry mouth as a side effect include:

- Antihistamines
- Antidepressants
- Antianxiety medications
- Blood pressure and heart medications, such as angiotensin-converting enzyme (ACE) inhibitors, calcium channel blockers, beta-blockers, heart rhythm medications, and diuretics
- Antinausea medications
- Antidiarrheal medications
- Antacids
- Parkinson's disease medications

- Alzheimer's disease medications
- Antiseizure medications
- Antispasm medications
- Antipsychotics
- Narcotic painkillers
- Isotretinoin to treat acne
- Scopolamine to prevent motion sickness

If you are experiencing severe dry mouth, check with your doctor to see if another medication might work better for you. If that is not possible, you will have to try to make some changes in your life to counteract the effect. Here are a few tactics that have worked for my patients:

- Sip a sugarless drink or water during the day.
- Reduce or skip drinking caffeinated beverages and alcohol, both of which have diuretic effects that contribute to dry mouth.
- Suck on sugarless candy or chew sugarless gum—stevia is the sugar substitute sweetener of choice—to promote saliva production.
- Stop smoking, if you haven't already. Using tobacco will dry out your mouth even more.
- Avoid spicy or salty foods, which can be painful in a dry mouth.
- Use a humidifier.

SWOLLEN GUMS

Some medications can cause gum tissue to build up, a condition known as gingival overgrowth. Gums can become so swollen that the tissue begins to grow over the teeth, increasing your risk of periodontal disease. Swollen gum tissue creates a favorable environment for anaerobic bacteria. Medications that can cause the gums to enlarge include:

- Immunosuppressant drugs such as cyclosporine, which is used to prevent transplant rejection
- Blood pressure medications, specifically calcium channel blockers
- Antiseizure medications

If you are on these medications and your gums are enlarging, you must pay meticulous attention to how you clean your teeth. You will need to brush and floss with extra care to avoid irritating swollen gum tissue. Consult with your dentist for tips on gentle oral care. You certainly do not want to apply a chemical-packed toothpaste to sensitive gums.

ABNORMAL BLEEDING

If you are taking blood thinners, such as aspirin and anticoagulants, your aim is to slow down the blood's clotting ability in order to help prevent heart attacks and stroke. But blood thinners can contribute to heavy bleeding from your gums, especially during oral surgery.

Tell your dentist you are taking blood thinners so that steps can be taken to minimize bleeding during periodontal work or oral surgery. When brushing and flossing, use a soft toothbrush with gentle motions to reduce bleeding.

FUNGAL INFECTIONS

Some asthma inhalers can lead to oral candidiasis, also known as thrush or yeast infection. Rinsing your mouth and gargling with water after using the inhaler will prevent this infection. If the problem persists, your dentist might prescribe antifungal lozenges or mouthwash to clear up the condition.

TASTE CHANGES

A medication can sometimes alter your sense of taste, causing a metallic, salty, or bitter taste in your mouth or change the taste of what you eat. Elderly patients who are taking several medications commonly experience this symptom. Many drugs have been linked to taste changes, among them:

- Chemotherapy drugs, including methotrexate and doxorubicin
- Antihistamines
- Antibiotics, such as ampicillin and tetracycline
- Antifungals
- Antipsychotics
- Asthma medicines
- Blood pressure medications
- Blood thinners
- Cholesterol-lowering drugs
- Corticosteroids
- Diabetes medications
- Diuretics
- Glaucoma medications
- Gout medications
- Nitroglycerin patches for the heart
- Iron-deficiency anemia medications
- Muscle relaxers
- Parkinson's disease medications
- Rheumatoid arthritis treatments
- Antiseizure medications
- Thyroid medications

- Transplant rejection drugs
- Nicotine skin patches
- Amphetamines

If food just doesn't taste the same, check with your doctor to see if another medication will not have a taste-altering effect.

INFLAMMATION OF THE MOUTH'S LINING

When the moist tissue lining the mouth, the mucous membrane, becomes inflamed, the condition is called mucositis. Certain chemotherapy drugs can cause mucositis, particularly if you drink alcohol, are dehydrated, smoke, do not take good care of your teeth and gums, and have diabetes, kidney disease, or HIV.

If you develop inflammation or the soft tissues in your mouth become discolored, talk to your dentist about designing a dental care regimen to reduce any discomfort you may be experiencing.

SORES IN YOUR MOUTH

Mouth ulcers or canker sores are open sores that occur on the tongue or in the mouth. They are known as craters because each ulcer has a hole in the middle, a break in the mucous membrane that lines the mouth. Drugs that can cause mouth sores to develop include:

- Many chemotherapy medications
- Aspirin
- Penicillin
- Streptomycin
- Antiseizure medicine
- Sulfonamide antibiotics used to treat ulcerative colitis
- Oral contraceptives
- Immunosuppressive agents

Discuss with your doctor whether alternative medications can be substituted for what you are taking. Your dentist can recommend a dental care regimen that will avoid irritation and speed healing. You should start by using toxin-free toothpaste and alcohol-free mouthwash.

TOOTH DISCOLORATION

Sixty years ago, in the 1950s, we discovered that the use of the antibiotic tetracycline during pregnancy could lead to brown discoloration in children's teeth. Some of the tetracycline taken settles into the calcium that the body uses to build teeth, causing the teeth that grow to have a yellow tone. When exposed to sunlight, those teeth turn brown.

If taken after teeth are formed, tetracycline does not discolor teeth. Discoloration only occurs when the medicine is taken before the primary and secondary teeth come in. Tetracycline and related antibiotics are not recommended during pregnancy or in children under the age of eight, whose teeth are still developing.

Other medicines cause staining on existing teeth. The list of medicines that follows can cause brown, yellow-brown, or gray discoloration in teeth:

- Augmentin (amoxicillin-clavulanate), an antibiotic that treats a number of bacterial infections
- Tetracycline, used to treat acne and some respiratory infections
- Doxycycline, a tetracycline antibiotic used to treat acne
- Chlorhexidine, an antiseptic/disinfectant used to clean skin after an injury or before surgery and injections
- Too much fluoride found in some chewable vitamins, toothpastes, and mouthwash

Taking some drugs may result in a green or blue-green color:

* Cipro (ciprofloxacin), an antibiotic
* Minocycline, an antibiotic related to tetracycline

Black teeth:

* Iron salts taken orally for anemia

If you are planning to get pregnant, avoid taking tetracycline. When you need an antibiotic, discuss your concerns about tooth discoloration with your doctor to avoid taking an antibiotic that appears on this list. If you have noticed some discoloration, consult with your dentist about the situation before it becomes irreversible.

BONE LOSS

A number of medications can lead to the loss of bone that supports your teeth. Drugs used to treat osteoporosis can affect the jawbone, causing a rare condition called osteonecrosis of the jawbone.

The symptoms of bone loss include painful, swollen gums or jaw, loose teeth, jaw numbness, fluid in the gums and jaw, a heavy feeling in the jaw.

The drugs that can promote loss of bone that supports teeth are:

* Corticosteroids such as prednisone
* Antiepileptic drugs

Drugs that cause osteonecrosis:

* Biphophonates used to treat osteoporosis

Let your dentist know if you are taking any of these drugs. If you are taking a drug for osteoporosis long term, your dentist may prescribe an antibiotic or nonsteroidal anti–inflammatory drug to slow bone loss.

TOOTH DECAY

Remember the immortal line "A spoonful of sugar helps the medicine go down" from *Mary Poppins*? That may be true, but the sugar in medicine can decay your teeth and those of your children. If you are taking long-term medications, check the ingredients for sugar. You are at a greater risk of developing tooth decay when you use sweetened medications. Sugar is often an ingredient in:

- Liquid medications
- Cough drops
- Vitamins
- Antacids

Consider taking sugar-free medications or changing from liquid to tablet form. To lessen sugar's effect, take the medication with a meal if allowed. After you take a sugary medication, rinse out your mouth with water.

Children are particularly vulnerable, because they often take syrupy medications, such as cough or cold medicine, which leave a sweet, sticky residue in their mouths. Make sure your children rinse with water every time they take sugar-loaded medications.

I wanted to cover some problematic side effects of medications to help you be more aware of yet another factor that contributes to the state of your oral health. If you notice changes in your mouth, review the medications you are taking longterm and those you have taken for a limited time to deal with an illness. Discuss any changes you observe with your doctor and your dentist and try to determine if the medications you are taking have influenced your oral ecosystem.

Remembering that the mouth⇔body connection is bidirectional, you will realize that the powerful medications you are taking for one condition can disrupt the balance in your mouth, which will affect the rest of your body. You need to break this feedback loop if you want to stay healthy. The relationships among the various systems in your body are complex. So many factors are at play that affect your body's healthy balance. Managing the medications you take with your physician and your dentist is one factor you can control. Whether you change medications, treat the conditions a medication causes in your mouth, or take steps to minimize the drug's effect, you can take action to protect and restore your oral health.

"SILVER" FILLINGS ARE FAR FROM PRECIOUS METAL

The last frontier in detoxing your mouth involves your "silver" fillings. Since amalgam fillings are not bonded to your teeth, they do not strengthen teeth that have been weakened from tooth decay. A tooth restored with amalgam is not a strongly reinforced tooth. It is common to see cracks in your teeth caused by the way the tooth is wedged with a metal filling. In addition, amalgam fillings require removal of healthy tooth structure in order for the amalgam material to perform satisfactorily. But I have held back on the really bad news.

The amalgam that most dentists use to fill patients' teeth is a mixture of metal that is silver in color. Dental amalgam is composed of liquid mercury mixed with powdered alloy metals, including silver, tin, and copper. A full 50 percent of this mix is mercury, a heavy metal and neurotoxin, the most toxic naturally occurring substance on earth. Mercury is used to bind the alloy particles together.

Amalgam is not stable after it is implanted in your teeth. According to the International Academy of Oral Medicine and Toxicology (IAOMT), amalgam fillings release a toxic mercury vapor that travels throughout your body. When the vapor is inhaled, mercury is absorbed through your lungs. Exposure to mercury vapor has been associated with bad effects in the brain and the kidneys.

Your brain is a primary target for heavy metals. Mercury vapor readily passes through your cell membranes, across your blood-brain barrier, and into your central nervous system, causing immunological, neurological, and psychological problems, including depression, anxiety, irritability, and memory loss. Mercury has been associated with neurodegeneration that leads to Alzheimer's disease and dementia. Does it make sense to implant such a toxic substance anywhere near your bloodstream and an inch from your brain?

At the same time, mercury leaches into your saliva and is swallowed, making its way down your digestive tract. On its journey through your body, mercury causes inflammation and affects your immune system's ability to eliminate the toxin. Certain factors increase the amount of mercury that leaches into the body, including the number of fillings you have, how old the fillings are, how acidic your diet is, and whether you grind your teeth. Mercury from your fillings can build up in your body, which is called bioaccumulation, the steadily increasing concentration of a chemical in organs and tissues.

Continued pressure from chewing eventually can cause filling materials and the teeth around them to crack. The edges of a filling can become detached from the tooth. Bacteria can then enter around the filling and cause further tooth decay. Aside from possible infections, mercury vapor can leach directly into your gums and bloodstream.

Cheryl was referred to me by her fertility doctor, who was first concerned with her dental condition, which included a mouth full of failing amalgam fillings with decay. She claimed she had these mercury-laden fillings from a young girl. We developed a schedule to safely remove and replace them with new BPA-free composite fillings and ceramic crowns. She then began a systemic detox for all heavy metals including mercury. Months after completion, she returned on a checkup visit beaming. She was pregnant at last.

THE SMOKING TOOTH

Roger Eichmann, DDS, held an extracted tooth containing an old amalgam filling in a miner's black light, a mercury emission light. He dipped the tooth in water heated to 100 degrees F to simulate the mild increase in temperature that results from tooth grinding, chewing, or drinking hot liquids. The smoke that visibly emerged from the tooth was the shadow of mercury vapor. You can see a video of the steady emission of mercury vapor from a filling that had been in someone's mouth for years on YouTube under the title "The Smoking Tooth" or "Smoking Teeth." They say one picture is worth a thousand words. Seeing that vapor is a good motivator to replace those "silver" fillings.

Studies have shown that after ten minutes of chewing gum, the mercury concentration in air of the mouth does not change in subjects who do not have amalgam fillings, but for those who do, mercury increases eight to tenfold and remains elevated for at least ninety minutes.

Austria, Germany, and Canada have restricted the use of dental amalgam mercury fillings, especially in children and pregnant women. In 2008, Norway, Sweden, and Denmark each banned dental amalgam mercury fillings altogether. I only hope that when dentists remove amalgam fillings they use proper mercury exposure protection for their patients, staff, and themselves.

Have You Been Exposed to Too Much Mercury from Amalgam Fillings?

The International Academy of Oral Medicine and Toxology (IAOMT) has listed the following signs that can indicate you are suffering from mercury exposure from your fillings:

* Anxiety
* Balance issues
* Bleeding gums
* Burning, tingling of lips
* Concentration problems
* Depression
* Drowsiness
* Insomnia
* Irritability
* Lethargy
* Memory loss
* Metallic taste
* Muscle weakness
* Nausea
* Numbness and tingling in hands, feet, fingers, and face
* Ringing ears
* Speech impairment
* Stiff neck and shoulder pain
* Tremors in hands, feet, fingers, eyes

As you can see from this long and varied list—each and every symptom can interfere with your feeling of well-being, giving you a general sense of malaise. The effect of amalgam fillings can persist as long as mercury remains in your mouth.

REPLACING AMALGAM FILLINGS

Much safer BPA-free composite filling materials are now in use made of quartz or glass in resin. This new filling material has cosmetic advantages, because they are close in color to natural teeth. Other restorative options are porcelain, ceramic, and gold restorations that strengthen the teeth without potential long-term health risks.

Extreme caution is required when amalgam fillings are removed. Taking out fillings with a high-speed dental bur creates a cloud of tiny particles you can inhale into your lungs, where the particles break down and the mercury is absorbed systemically. This mercury exposure can be as much as a hundred times greater than from mercury vapor. I use a very rigorous protocol at Rejuvenation Dentistry for safe amalgam removal.

This is what we do to protect our patients and ourselves from mercury:

1. Patients take activated charcoal ten to fifteen minutes before the procedure begins, because the charcoal can bind small particles of swallowed mercury, allowing them to pass through the body without harm.
2. We have a special air filtration system to keep the air pure in the entire office.
3. An air filtering system is placed close to the patient's mouth for extra protection.
4. During the removal process, water and air cool the filling to reduce the mercury vapor the filling releases.
5. The tip of a powerful suction system is placed very close to the filling during the removal process. Using a high-volume evacuator this way minimizes my patients' exposure to amalgam particles and mercury vapor.
6. Our patients use a nasal hood through which they breathe pure oxygen. An alternative source of air is protective

while the filling is being removed. We advise patients to breathe only through the nose to avoid inhaling mercury particles or fumes.

7. I use a rubber dam to isolate the tooth being worked on. Despite the protection, mercury can penetrate the latex of the dam.

8. I remove the amalgam filling by cutting it into chunks. Chunking involves less drilling and avoids creating fine particles. I can then remove pieces of amalgam with suction or a hand instrument.

9. We vacuum patients' mouths thoroughly and have them rinse to cleanse the mouth of amalgam particles and residual mercury vapor—no swallowing allowed. After a fifteen-second rinse, the next step is to gargle far back in the throat and spit into the sink.

10. We remove and dispose of the protective covering patients wear and clean their faces and necks thoroughly.

11. When the removal is complete and the new filling is in place, I advise my patients to follow up with antioxidant nutritional support, namely the supplements chlorella, a fresh water, single cell, green algae, available in capsule and powder form, which neutralizes heavy metals such as mercury; selenium, a trace element; and Vitamin C to boost the immune system and fight infection.

If you are going to the trouble and expense of removing your amalgam fillings, you want to make certain that your dentist is taking the right precautions to protect you from mercury released in the process.

In this chapter, I have focused on factors that affect the condition of your mouth that you can do something about. From minimizing your exposure to toxins to using a toothpaste that keeps your oral microbiome in balance, from being aware of how medications can affect the climate in your mouth to the potential health hazard of "silver" amalgam fillings, this chapter prepares you for the first stage in cleaning up your act.

A new patient, Ivan, had a mouth full of ill-fitting, all metal crowns. He reported that shortly after the work was done in Russia, he began suffering from severe "burning" headaches and major digestive problems. Despite many medical consultations and tests, no one suspected his dental work could be the problem.

After removing the old metal crowns, which had recurrent decay, I had the metal analyzed and was shocked to find it was almost 70 percent nickel, a toxic-heavy metal and known carcinogen. It was no surprise that he was suffering painful symptoms with so much toxic material in his mouth.

When the old crowns were safely removed, Ivan began a systemic detox protocol and reported his digestion improved almost immediately and his headaches subsided almost completely.

The following chapter gives you guidelines for how to eat to reduce inflammation. My Triple A Diet is not about weight loss, though you very well might lose a few pounds when you change the way you eat. This is not a diet you go on for the course of the 28-Day Program and then return to your old eating habits. What I prescribe is a fundamental change in the food you eat for life. Chapter 7 details the way to eat to avoid acidity throughout your body and to reduce health-destroying inflammation.

Chapter Seven

The Triple A Diet

Anti-inflammatory, Alkalizing, Antioxidant

My Triple A Diet, which I also call A-List Diet, is designed to get inflammation under control. I don't have to remind you that inflammation is at the root of most disease. The good news is that you can fight inflammation with a diet that puts out the fire by making your body less acidic and giving it the antioxidant support it needs to fight free radicals.

In general, I recommend an alkaline-promoting/low-acidic diet. The standard American diet, also known by the appropriate acronym SAD, is far too high in acid-promoting processed foods, bad fats, and artificial sweeteners, and low on fresh vegetables, which are alkaline. Since sugar and carbs are acidic and cause breakdowns in the ecology of your mouth, my diet is low on simple carbohydrates. Emotional stress, toxic overload, and immune reactions can shift your pH from a healthy, slightly alkaline state to an acidic one. The first focus of the Triple A Diet concerns the role your pH level has in your overall health and provides lists of alkalizing foods and supplements. This chapter covers inflammatory foods that stoke the fire and what to eat to counter inflammation, including spices and supplements.

Eating antioxidant-rich foods, containing Vitamins A, B, C, and E; coenzyme Q-10; pantothenic acid; and quercetin, is essential when your immune system is on "high alert" as a result of stress and inflammation. I explain how free radicals are formed and the damage they can do to your body. The chapter includes a list of foods with antioxidant qualities and those to avoid. I also suggest the vitamins you need to take daily to support your anti-inflammatory lifestyle.

Let's begin with the fundamental do's and don'ts for a way to eat that will promote balance in your body.

THE ROOTS OF THE TRIPLE A DIET

One of my heroes is Weston A. Price, an American dentist in the first half of the twentieth century, who was a visionary and a thought leader, way ahead of his time. During the 1930s, he traveled around the world on an anthropological mission: to identify the factors that led to good dental health. He studied indigenous people from North and South America, African tribes, South Sea Islanders, New Zealand Maori, Australian aborigines, and people in remote villages in Switzerland and the Hebrides. He studied their dental and physical health, analyzed their diets, and did follow-up research on nutrition. During his travels, he found that native people had terrific, straight teeth, free from decay, and that the people were resistant to disease. He published his findings in a book called *Nutrition and Physical Degeneration*, which is still used decades later. He found that when people chose convenience foods over traditional nourishment, their health degenerates.

In comparison to the American diet in the 1930s, isolated native people consumed at least four times the water-soluble vitamins, calcium, and other minerals. Their diets contained at least ten times the fat-soluble Vitamins A and D from animal foods, such as butter, fish, eggs, shellfish, organ meats, and animal fats. Think of how we eat today. Those foods came to be considered unhealthy, because of the fear surrounding high-cholesterol levels.

This narrow focus ignores the fact that Vitamins A and D support mineral and protein absorption and use, which are essential for good health. Dr. Price went on to discover another fat-soluble nutrient, which is now called Vitamin K_2, found in fish livers, shellfish, organ meats, and butter made from the milk of grass-fed cows. If you would like to read more about his findings, have a look at the Weston A. Price Foundation website, http://www .westonaprice.org.

His dietary guidelines, which he began publishing at the beginning of the twentieth century, demonstrate that he was prescient and had a profound understanding of what the body needs to stay in balance. Most of his discoveries have become mainstream today. I have adapted some of his basic ideas in the Triple A Diet. Many of these points go against the principles of trendy diets that tend to limit consumption of whole categories of food.

1. **Eat whole, natural foods.** Eat only foods that will spoil, but eat them before they do. Staying away from the high sugar, salt, and fat content in processed foods is a big move in fighting inflammation.
2. **Eat natural, organically raised meat, including fish, seafood, poultry, beef, lamb, game, organ meats, and eggs.** You want to avoid the hormones and antibiotics now used in conventionally raised meat, fish, poultry, and eggs.
3. **Eat whole, organic milk products from pasture-fed cows**, such as whole yogurt, whole cheeses, and fresh and sour cream. Forget about fat free. The fat is nourishing, and if you remove it, you are left with simple carbs. Conventionally raised cows and goats are given hormones so that they produce more milk.
4. **Use extra virgin olive oil, expeller-expressed sesame and flaxseed oil, and the tropical oils, coconut and palm**. These are healthy fats.

5. **Eat fresh fruits and vegetables, preferably organic**, in salads and soups. To prepare, lightly steam or roast the vegetables with a little olive oil.

6. **Soak nuts and edible seeds overnight in water**. Sprouting, as this process is called, makes seeds and nuts more easily digestible and neutralizes phytic acid, one of the antinutrients, which can block calcium, zinc, magnesium, iron, and copper absorption.

7. **Include enzyme-enhanced lacto-fermented vegetables, fruits, beverages, and condiments on a regular basis**, such as sauerkraut, dill pickles, and kombucha. The group of recipes that begin on page 234 will show you how easy it is to prepare lacto-fermented foods.

8. **Prepare homemade bone broth** and use liberally in soups and sauces. You can find bone broth recipes on page 246.

9. **Use herb teas and coffee substitutes in moderation.**

10. **Use filtered water for cooking and drinking.**

11. **Use unrefined Celtic Sea Salt and a variety of herbs and spices.**

12. **Make your own salad dressing using extra virgin olive oil.**

13. **Use natural sweeteners in moderation**, such as raw honey, maple syrup, and green stevia powder.

14. **Cook only in stainless steel, cast iron, glass, or good-quality enamel.** Avoid aluminum and nonstick surfaces that contain fluorinated chemicals.

You might not be familiar with some of the points on this list. Phytic acid, lacto-fermented food, and bone broths may be new to you. Knowing how they affect you and changing your eating habits accordingly will help keep your microbiome healthy and assure that you are not mineral deficient.

Biggest Nutritional Influences on Your Oral Health

According to Weston Price, three main factors have the biggest effect on your oral health:

* Consuming sufficient minerals in your diet.
* Consuming fat-soluble vitamins, specifically Vitamins A, D, E, and K.
* The bioavailability of these nutrients and how well your body absorbs them, which means reducing or neutralizing phytic acid in your diet.

WHY PHYTIC ACID IS IN THE NO-FLY ZONE

Phytic acid or phytate, found in plant seeds, is the main storage form of phosphorus in seeds. All edible seeds, grains, legumes, and nuts contain it, and small amounts are found in roots and tubers. In grains, most of the phytic acid is found in the bran. This warning conflicts with our current obsession with eating only whole grains, in which the bran is intact and loaded with phytic acid. The problem is that phytic acid impairs the absorption of iron, zinc, magnesium, and calcium, which can contribute to mineral deficiencies that affect your teeth.

Avoiding all foods containing phytic acid is not practical. For example, nuts like almonds are nutritious and healthy. Preparing grains, nuts, seeds, and beans makes a difference. When seeds sprout, phytic acid is degraded and the phosphorus is released for the seedlings' use. You can reduce the amount of phytic acid in the food you eat in three easy ways:

* **Soaking** grains, nuts, and legumes in water overnight.
* **Sprouting or germinating** seeds, grains, and legumes, which degrades phytate germination.

- **Fermenting** foods, which forms organic acids that cause phytate to break down. I go into this method in more detail in the next section.

Not only will taking this extra step keep your phytic acid intake under control, but it will also make these foods easier to digest.

WHAT IS LACTO-FERMENTED FOOD AND WHY SHOULD YOU EAT IT?

If you are like my patients, you probably do not know what lacto-fermentation is and wonder why incorporating lacto-fermented food into your diet is important. Lacto-fermentation has been used to preserve food long before we had ways to keep our food cold to avoid spoilage, artificial preservatives, or enough heat to can food. Modern methods to preserve food—including a host of chemicals—deaden and denature food. Lacto-fermentation keeps food alive, making nutrients more available and foods enzyme-rich and pro-biotic. Just a little liquid whey or salt added to cooked or uncooked vegetables and fruit produce probiotic *Lactobacillus* bacterial cultures. These friendly bacteria convert starches and sugars in vegetables and fruits to lactic acid, a natural preservative.

Lacto-fermentation allows good bacteria to flourish. That's right, pickling vegetables and fruits in this way creates probiotic foods. If you have eaten sauerkraut or pickles, you have experienced lacto-fermented food. From Old-Fashioned Dill Pickled Green Beans to Salsa with a Kick, you will find a number of recipes and instructions for making these microbiome-protecting foods beginning on page 234.

BONE BROTH

Bone broth is the latest diet trend, but your grandmother most likely made broth all the time. In every four-star restaurant, a large stockpot simmers on a back burner, because freshly made broth or stock has great flavor and endless culinary uses. Nutrient-rich bone broth is also a powerful health tonic that is high in calcium, magnesium, and phosphorus, all of which are wonderful for bone and tooth health. Sipping on bone broth is great for healing teeth and gums. Bone broth is soothing and boosts the immune system. It can be made from the bones of beef, lamb, poultry, or fish with vegetables and spices. You can sip on the broth anytime during the day or use the broth in soups, stews, gravies, sauces, and reductions. Chapter 15 introduces you to the joy of making your own bone broth.

DR. GERRY'S WHAT NOT TO EAT

If you want to feel great, boost your energy, and put the brakes on aging, you have to get the junk out of the trunk, as I like to say. You have to be willing to eliminate certain foods from your diet, or at least significantly reduce your intake of these foods. I don't want you to find the list daunting. Once you begin eating healthier foods, you will see and feel a difference. Your increased sense of well-being will motivate you to keep it up.

Before you start the program, go through your kitchen cabinets and refrigerator and get rid of the foods that appear on the taboo list or put those items aside so that you will not be tempted to fall off the wagon. If you feel you are wasting food, you might want to delay starting the program until you have gone through your supply of no-nos, though my attitude is: Why put it off? The sooner you start, the sooner you will feel better than ever. Say good-bye to:

- Processed foods including cakes, cookies, crackers, frozen dinners, sweet and soft drinks—staples of the standard American diet.

- Refined sugars. Sugar goes by many names on labels. Any ingredient that ends in "ose" is a refined sweetener. Fruit juices count.
- Anything made with white flour—such as bread, rolls, and other baked goods, pasta, and don't forget simple carbohydrates such as white rice and white potatoes.
- Hydrogenated or partially hydrogenated fats and oils, which are solid—think trans-fats.
- All industrial polyunsaturated vegetable oils made from soy, corn, safflower, canola, or cottonseed.
- Foods fried or cooked in polyunsaturated oils or partially hydrogenated vegetable oils, which means fast food.
- Low-fat or skim milk, powdered milk, or imitation milk.
- Factory-farmed eggs, meats, and fish. Eat free-range, organic, or wild caught.
- Cold cuts and sausage that are highly processed.
- Canned, sprayed, waxed, and irradiated fruits and vegetables.
- Genetically modified foods (GMOs) found in most corn, canola, and soy products.
- Artificial food additives such as preservatives, coloring, and MSG, which are found in most ready-made soups, sauces, and condiments.
- Caffeine—or at least keep your consumption to a minimum.
- Aluminum, found in baking powder, commercial salt, antacids, and cookware.
- Unfiltered fluoridated water.
- Synthetic vitamins and foods that contain taboo ingredients.
- Microwave ovens, because they change the chemical structure of food.

Now that the foundation for eating for balance is established, it is time to take a look at active ways you can fight inflammation.

THE SEA INSIDE

Fluids are responsible for 70 percent of your body weight, which is the same percentage of water to land on earth. The fluids in your body are acid, neutral, or alkaline. Your stomach has the highest acidity to aid in digestion and to protect against opportunistic microbes. Your skin is acidic to serve as a barrier to the environment and to protect against microbial overgrowth. In order for all the systems in your body to function well, your body fluids have to border on being alkaline.

Your pH balance indicates how acidic or alkaline your body is. The range from acidic to alkaline is measured on a scale of 0 to 14. The higher your pH level is, the more alkaline the balance in your internal fluids; the lower your pH, the more acidic. Purified water has a neutral pH balance of 7.0. A pH level less than 7 is considered acidic; greater than 7 is base or alkaline.

Your pH controls intercellular activity, regulates your digestive system, and determines how your body uses enzymes, minerals, and vitamins. When your body converts food to energy, the processes of digestion and absorption create by-products that can be acidic. The standard modern diet, complete with coffee, processed foods, commercially raised meat, dairy products that are not organic, and a lack of fresh produce promotes excess acidity. Stress can make your body acidic as well. When acid levels in your body become too high, it is difficult for you to excrete the acid to return to balance. An acidic environment can cause tooth decay. When your internal environment is acidic, the imbalance can lead to degeneration and disease, because the body scavenges vital minerals from your bones and teeth in an attempt to neutralize the acid pH.

The symptoms of pH imbalance can be subtle. You may feel fatigued and lethargic. The symptoms associated with having an acid body include:

Weight gain
Loss of elasticity in skin

Loss of vitality

Joint pain

Aching muscles

Stomach ache

Ulcers

Nausea

Urinary tract problems

Kidney stones

Constipation

Immune deficiency

Gout

Constriction of blood vessels

Osteopenia

Osteoporosis

Circulatory and vascular weakness

Many of these serious symptoms are hidden and you won't discover them until you're in danger.

Making different food choices can reduce these symptoms to prevent you from experiencing them, because what you eat affects your pH. If you want the microbial communities throughout your body to be balanced, you have to reduce the acidity in your body. The good news is that you can make your internal pH more alkaline by changing your diet.

ALKALINE NUTRITION

Food shapes the pH environment in which your cells live. Good nutrition helps to build extracellular fluid that is slightly alkaline. An alkaline or base environment allows cells to absorb nutrients and discharge toxins, and promotes the proper function of your organs, including kidneys, liver, large intestine, and skin. The best way to build your body's reserves of buffering minerals, including calcium, sodium, potassium, and magnesium, is to eat an alkalizing diet with mineral and vitamin supplements. The ideal balance is 80 percent alkaline-forming foods and 20 percent acid-forming foods.

These are some steps you can take to reduce the acidity in your body:

- Eat fruits and vegetables that are rich in enzymes.
- Avoid white sugar.
- Eat less meat. I suggest no more than three servings of red meat per week.
- Stick to extra virgin olive oil and coconut oil.
- Use fresh lemon, which is one of the most alkaline fruits. Try hot lemon water in the morning and make lemon your favorite condiment.
- Eat more sprouted nuts, seeds, and grains.

As a quick reference, I am including two tables that will show you what to eat and what to cut back on.

Eat More—80 percent of your diet should be composed of these foods.

Highly Alkaline	Moderately Alkaline	Mildly Alkaline
pH 9.5 alkaline water	Avocado	Artichokes
Himalayan salt	Beets	Asparagus
Cucumber	Basil	Brussels sprouts
Kale	Black pepper	Cauliflower
Kelp and sea vegetables	Cabbage	Carrot
Spinach	Celery	Eggplant
Parsley	Chives	Leeks
Broccoli	Collard greens	New potatoes
Sprouts	Coriander	Peas
Green drinks	Endive	Pumpkin

Highly Alkaline	Moderately Alkaline	Mildly Alkaline
All sprouted beans and seeds	Garlic	Squash
	Ginger	Grapefruit
	Green beans	Coconut
	Lettuce	Pomegranate
	Mustard greens	Rhubarb
	Okra	Buckwheat
	Onion	Lentils
	Radish	Tofu
	Red onion	Almond milk
	Rocket/arugula	Goat milk
	Tomato	Herbs and spices
	Lemon	Avocado oil
	Lime	Olive oil
	Butter beans	Coconut oil
	Soybeans	Flaxseed oil
	White haricot beans	
	Chia seeds	
	Quinoa	

Eat Less—No more than 20 percent of your diet should be composed of these foods.

Neutral/Mildly Acidic	Moderately Acidic	Highly Acidic
Black beans	Fresh, natural juice	Alcohol
Chickpeas	Ketchup	Coffee
Kidney beans and other beans	Mayonnaise	Black tea
Seitan	Butter	Unsweetened fruit juice
Cantaloupe	Apple	Cocoa
Nectarine	Apricot	Honey
Plum	Banana	Jam
Sweet cherries	Blackberry	Jelly
Watermelon	Blueberry	Mustard
Amaranth	Cranberry	Miso

Neutral/Mildly Acidic	*Moderately Acidic*	*Highly Acidic*
Millet	Grapes	Soy sauce
Oats/oatmeal	Guava	Vinegar
Spelt	Mango	Yeast
Soybeans	Orange	Dried fruit
Rice/soy/hemp protein	Peach	Beef
Freshwater wild fish	Papaya	Chicken
Rice and soy milk	Pineapple	Eggs
Brazil nuts	Strawberry	Farmed fish
Pecans	Goat cheese	Pork
Hazelnuts	Brown rice	Shellfish
Sunflower oil	Rye bread	Cheese
Grape seed oil	Wheat	Dairy
	Whole meal bread	Artificial sweeteners
	Wild rice	Syrup
	Ocean fish	Mushrooms

Now that you know how to eat to reduce acidity, you are ready to take on those free radicals you have been hearing about.

STOPPING FREE RADICALS IN THEIR TRACKS

Antioxidants counter oxidation, a normal chemical process as the body metabolizes oxygen. When the body is healthy, oxygen metabolism is very efficient. Only 1 to 2 percent of cells get damaged and turned into free radicals. Free radicals are exactly what they sound like. They are unstable molecules that interact aggressively with other molecules and create abnormal cells. In stable molecules, pairs of electrons ring the nucleus. Free radicals have an unmated electron, which is looking to hook up with another electron to form a pair. When free radicals steal an electron from a neighboring molecule to complete the pair, the attacked molecule becomes a free radical. This action can set off a chain reaction, a form of inflammation that damages cell structures and DNA. The chain reaction is called oxidative stress, which happens when the body's supply of antioxidants is not sufficient to handle and neutralize the free radicals produced by oxidation. The same process occurs when metal rusts or when a slice of apple turns brown.

External toxins also create free radicals. Drinking alcohol, smoking, and sunbathing can promote free radical production. Air pollution, infection, and exposure to toxins of all sorts throws off the balance in your body and pushes the body toward oxidative stress. Free radicals set the course for disease by breaking down tissue and weakening the immune system. When free radicals are out of control, they accelerate aging and contribute to the development of chronic illnesses such as Alzheimer's, Parkinson's, cancer, and cardiovascular disease to name a few.

As you age, your natural defenses against free radical rampages become less effective. A high level of antioxidants in your diet can help to prevent age-related diseases.

ANTIOXIDANTS

The most effective way to combat free radicals is to consume foods high in antioxidants rather than relying on supplements. For example, raspberries and strawberries contain ellagic acid, which is not well absorbed in supplement form. Let's look at a number of antioxidants and their nutritional sources.

> **Vitamin C:** bell peppers, berries, broccoli, kiwi fruit, mangoes, oranges and other citrus fruit, spinach
> **Vitamin E:** avocados, nuts, especially almonds, olive oil, seeds
> **Allium sulphur compounds:** garlic, leeks, onions
> **Anthocyanins** (found in blue and purple food): blueberries, eggplant, plums, pomegranates, raspberries, red cabbage
> **Beta-carotene, which creates Vitamin A:** apricots, carrots, mangoes, parsley, pumpkin, spinach
> **Catechins:** red wine, tea
> **Copper:** lean meat, legumes, milk, nuts, seafood

Cryptoxanthins: mangoes, pumpkin, red peppers

Flavonoids: apples, citrus fruits, green tea, onions, red wine, tea

Indoles: cruciferous vegetables, including broccoli, Brussels sprouts, cabbage, cauliflower

Lignans (found in high-fiber food): berries, broccoli, cashews, flaxseeds, kale, poppy seeds, sesame seeds, sunflower seeds, whole grains

Lutein: corn, dark leafy greens, including collard greens, kale, spinach

Lycopene (found in red fruits and vegetables): papaya, pink grapefruit, tomatoes, watermelon

Manganese: milk, lean meats, nuts, seafood

Polyphenols: oregano, thyme

Selenium: lean meat, seafood, whole grains

Zinc: lean meat, milk, nuts

SPICE UP YOUR LIFE

Recent research from Norway has found that dried herbs and spices are a very good source of dietary antioxidants. As little as ½ teaspoon of ground cloves contributes more antioxidants than ½ cup of blueberries or cranberries. Dried oregano also packs a powerful dose of antioxidants—½ teaspoon of dried oregano contains the antioxidants of ½ cup of sweet potatoes. Oregano has scored the highest in antioxidant activity of all tested herbs with three to twenty times higher antioxidant activity than all the herbs tested.

Top 10 Antioxidant Dried Herbs: cloves, allspice, cinnamon, rosemary, thyme, marjoram, saffron, oregano, tarragon, basil.

Top 6 Antioxidant Fresh Herbs: oregano, sage, peppermint, thyme, lemon balm, marjoram.

Before starting a new supplement regimen, always check with your physician to be certain you do not experience any undesired interactions with other medications you may be taking.

SUPPLEMENTS FOR THE MOUTH⇔BODY CONNECTION: THE 28-DAY CURATOLA CARE PROGRAM

Supplements are an important part of the 28-Day Curatola Care Program. They offer essential nutritional support for the repair and reversal of inflammation. With metabolomic formulations, which support cellular metabolisms, and herbalomic formulations, which provide specific support from botanicals and herbs, supplements help the body to "reboot" right down to a cellular level and tune up your epigenetics, which affects genetic expression. Combined with probiotic and prebiotic care for your mouth and gut microbiome, supplements help to prevent the propagation of various pathogens that wreak havoc throughout the body, fanning the flames of inflammation and creating poor digestion and dietary malabsorption.

Dietary supplements on the market today are often poorly sourced and synthetic, containing toxic ingredients. Many supplements are manufactured in a poorly controlled process. Reminiscent of the days of the traveling snake oil salesman, an alarming number of junk supplements, which are weakly regulated, sometimes make outlandish claims with no scientific data to back them up. There is a famous abdominal X-ray showing a completely undigested vitamin pill passing through the entire alimentary canal from the mouth to the colon totally intact with little absorption of the nutrients.

I have spent the good part of three decades researching dietary supplements of the highest-quality natural and organic ingredients that have gone through a rigorous research and development process with controlled clinical trials and published research. One such set of supplements I recommend in this section was developed by molecular biologist Shayne Morris Ph.D., founder of Nutribiome at Systemic Formulas in Ogden, Utah. These supplements are distributed by health care providers including chiropractors, nutritional consultants, naturopaths, acupuncturists, medical doctors, dentists, and veterinarians throughout the United States. Any health professional can order these supplements online at www.systemicformulas.com or by calling 800-445-4647. They are the best on the market, and I highly recommend them. The Curatola Care Program provides you with a schedule of what to take every day on each stage of the program.

This chapter has given you what you need to know about combating inflammation through your diet. My Curatola Care Program will ease you—step-by-step—into incorporating these important changes into the way you eat and help you make eating well a habit. By compiling all the nutritional information in this chapter, I have come up with a list of superfoods that are warriors in the fight against inflammation. I have taken these foods into account when I designed the meal plans to show you how easy it is to make these balancing foods a key component of your diet.

Chapter Eight

Dr. Gerry's Superfoods

As you can see from the lists of inflammation-fighting, anti-oxidant foods in the previous chapter, you have a cornucopia to choose from with the Triple A Diet. Healthy eating is a joy, not an ordeal. The Curatola Care Program will walk you through the changes to make in your eating habits to bring balance back to your body. The transition from processed junk food to a diet centered on fresh, whole food is easy to do. Once you shift from dead to living food, you will look and feel so much better that you might well lose your taste for food that is far from its original state. The excess of salt, sugar, and unhealthy fats in processed foods has addicted you to high flavor. When you stop getting a fix from convenience food—whether from a drive-through, a box, a can, or a bag—you will begin to appreciate the rich and subtle flavor of wholesome food in its natural state.

I have selected a baker's dozen of foods that are at the top of the food chain. These superfoods deliver peak nutrition and have far-reaching benefits. To convince you that these foods will do you a world of good, I have given you a comprehensive explanation of why I consider each a superfood. The meal plans and recipes that appear in Part 3 will show you how to enjoy these foods and make them the core of your diet.

ARCTIC CHAR: THE NEW SALMON

Arctic char is a tasty, pink, cold-water fish that is similar to salmon and trout. The fish's flavor is a balance between the mildly sweet, freshwater taste of trout and the more robust taste of salmon. It is light, moist, and firm in texture, and extremely versatile.

Until recently, char was caught in the cold waters of Iceland, Canada, Norway, Alaska, and Siberia and wasn't widely distributed beyond those regions. But fish farming has changed all that. Almost all of the Arctic char available in the United States is farmed in an environmentally friendly way. Farmed Arctic char is preferable to farmed salmon. Char is raised in tanks on shore, in contrast to salmon, which is usually raised in open netpens in coastal waters. The land-based tanks in which char is raised have excellent water quality control and protection against farmed fish escaping into the wild. In addition, onshore farming systems produce less pollution. Mercury contamination does not affect char raised on shore. Arctic char is on my list of superfoods because it is the purest and one of the most nutritious fish available. To add to its appeal, char is considerably less expensive than wild salmon.

Fish are an excellent source of protein, vitamins, minerals, and omega-3 fatty acids. Since it is an oily fish, Arctic char, in particular, has a high concentration of omega-3s. Omega-3 has been documented to reduce chronic inflammation, lower blood pressure, reduce plaque buildup in arteries, and may reduce the risk of developing some cancers. Marinating a piece of Arctic char or topping it with honey mustard and tossing it on the grill or in the broiler is all you have to do to prepare this healthy protein. A number of recipes are included in Chapter 15 to get you started. I like it better than salmon—it's more delicate.

AVOCADO: FRUIT WITH A DIFFERENCE

Avocado is the only fruit high in healthy fats, namely monoun-saturated fatty acids, also known as MUFA. The oleic acid in avocado is also the major component of olive oil. Avocado contains small amounts of sugar when compared with other fruits. The creamy, delicious fruit is packed with nutrients. A 3.5-ounce serving of avocado contains:

- Vitamin K: 26% [of the Recommended Dietary Allowance (RDA)]
- Folate: 20%
- Vitamin C: 17%
- Potassium: 14%
- Vitamin B_5: 14%
- Vitamin B_6: 13%
- Vitamin E: 10%
- Magnesium
- Manganese
- Copper
- Iron
- Zinc
- Phosphorous
- Potassium
- Vitamin A
- Vitamin B_1 (thiamine)
- Vitamin B_2 (riboflavin)
- Vitamin B_3 (niacin)

The carbohydrate content in avocado is mostly fiber, which not only helps to regulate appetite, but also feeds the friendly bacteria in the gut. Avocados increase the absorption of antioxidants from other foods and are high in antioxidants themselves, including the carotenoids, lutein and zeaxanthin, and the inflammation-fighting persenones A and B.

The health benefits of avocado are numerous. From reducing arthritis symptoms to protecting the liver from disease, from reducing bad breath and preventing oral cancer to improving your mood, avocado has the power to boost your health.

So bring on the guacamole!

CAULIFLOWER: THE TRENDY ANTI-INFLAMMATORY CRUSADER

Cauliflower is the new trendy vegetable, because there is so much you can do with it: eat it raw as a crudité, mash it for a satisfying potato substitute, roast a whole head, and season it liberally with spices such as turmeric. You can even make "Cauliflower Rice"— see pages 267–273 for recipes. My favorite is "Cauliflower Fried Rice," which satisfies many cravings.

Cauliflower is definitely not one of the white foods to avoid. It ranks among the top twenty foods on the Aggregate Nutrient Density Index (ANDI), which measures vitamin, mineral, and phytonutrient content, and antioxidant capacity in relation to caloric content.

The nutrient profile of 1 cup of cooked cauliflower is as impressive as its versatility:

- Vitamin C: 73% [of the RDA]
- Vitamin K: 19%
- Folate: 14%
- Vitamin B_5: 13% (pantothenic acid)
- Vitamin B_6: 12%
- Choline: 11%
- Fiber: 11%
- Omega-3 fats: 9%

- Manganese: 8%
- Phosphorus: 6%
- Biotin: 5%
- Potassium: 5%
- Vitamin B_2: 5%
- Vitamin B_1: 4%
- Magnesium: 3%
- Vitamin B_3: 3%

Cauliflower has not been the subject of as many studies as other cruciferous vegetables. I told you it's the hot new trend. Dozens of studies have linked eating cauliflower with cancer prevention, particularly cancer of the bladder, breast, colon, prostate, and ovaries. This vegetable contains indole-3-carbinol, a compound that may help to thwart the growth of cancer and to repair your DNA.

Cauliflower, like other cruciferous vegetables, also contains glucosinolates, which are phytonutrients that help to activate and regulate detoxification enzymes. The Vitamin C content as well as many phytonutrients gives cauliflower antioxidant benefits, which reduces oxidative stress and the inflammation that results from the free radical cascade.

An excellent source of Vitamin K, cauliflower is loaded with this most effective anti-inflammatory nutrient. Combined with its omega-3 content, cauliflower has cardiovascular benefits as well. The powerful anti-inflammatory nutrients found in cauliflower have sparked new research on how cauliflower reduces the risk of inflammation-related health problems, such as irritable bowel syndrome, obesity, type 2 diabetes, colitis, and rheumatoid arthritis.

Brussels sprouts and broccoli are great for you, too, but you can be much more creative in preparing cauliflower. Just look at the recipes that begin on page 267.

CELERY: MUCH MORE THAN A DIET FOOD

Most likely, you think of celery as a diet food with a lot of fiber and crunch. Recently, celery has been getting a lot of attention for antioxidant and anti-inflammatory effects. Rather than having simple sugars, which you want to avoid as much as possible, celery has nonstarchy polysaccharides that give it a unique structure. Apiuman is one of these nonstarchy polysaccharides that produce the anti-inflammatory benefits.

Celery contains well-known antioxidants such as flavonoids and Vitamin C, but scientists have identified at least a dozen other types of antioxidant nutrients that protect against oxidative damage to cells, blood vessels, and organ systems. Celery contains thirteen phytonutrients that are anti-inflammatory. It is high in Vitamins K, B_2, C, B_6, and A along with folate, potassium, manganese, pantothenic acid, copper, caladium, phosphorous, magnesium, and fiber.

Celery aids in digestion by restoring the proper level of hydrochloric acid in the stomach, which becomes out of balance from such drugs as Prilosec. Besides all the vitamins and vitality it has, celery helps to keep the body detoxed and at a proper pH.

Fresh celery, stored in the refrigerator, should be eaten within five to seven days. Though some nutrients appear to be stable in whole, refrigerated celery, a number of studies have shown greater losses of antioxidants after a week. It is advisable to wait to chop celery until just before you are adding it to a salad or cooked dish to preserve maximum nutrient value.

COCONUT: SCIENCE EXORCISED THE DEMONS

Coconuts and coconut-derived ingredients such as coconut oil, milk, and water have grown in popularity after a history of being demonized because of the high saturated fat content. Eighty-seven percent of the fatty acids in coconut are saturated. There has been a revolution in thinking about saturated fats. Many studies have shown that the notion that saturated fats clog the arteries is a myth. In fact, saturated fats have been shown to raise HDL (good) cholesterol and transform LDL (bad) cholesterol to a benign state. Coconut oil contains medium-chain triglycerides, not the long-chain fatty acids in other foods. The medium-chain fatty acids in coconut are metabolized differently. The fatty acids go straight to the liver from the digestive tract, where they are immediately converted to ketones, a quick source of energy, rather than being stored as fat.

About half of the medium-chain fatty acids in coconut consist of lauric acid. In the body, lauric acid is converted to monolaurin, an antiviral and antibacterial that destroys a variety of pathogenic bacteria, viruses, and fungi, including the dangerous *Staphylococcus aureus* and candida yeast.

Coconuts are rich in fiber; Vitamins C, B_1, B_3, B_5, and B_6; iron; selenium; sodium; calcium; magnesium; and phosphorous. The high levels of antioxidants in coconut oil reduce inflammation and arthritis pain. It also boosts the body's ability to absorb fat-soluble vitamins, calcium, and magnesium. If taken at the same time as omega-3 fatty acids, coconut oil will make the omega-3s twice as effective.

Coconut oil contributes to oral health as well. It has been used for centuries to cleanse the mouth of harmful bacteria and to help heal periodontal disease. If you want to heal your gums, try swishing coconut oil in your mouth three or four times a week for twenty minutes a day.

Aside from tasting great, coconut oil, milk, and cream fill you up. I put rich coconut cream in my morning shake to stay on top of the packed appointment schedule at the office. I can go all day without breaking for lunch. The side benefit for me has been weight loss without ever feeling deprived. This newly acknowledged superfood helps to bring your body back into balance while pleasing your palate.

FREE-RANGE, ORGANIC CHICKEN: CHICKEN SOUP REALLY DOES HEAL

Free-range or pastured chickens have some access to an outside area, which allows them to forage for grubs and plants in a natural environment. Do not be tricked by the label "cage-free," which means that chickens raised for meat were not kept in cages in a warehouse, but does not indicate that they were pastured. Look for the "Animal Welfare Approved" label or buy your poultry from a local farmer who guarantees the chickens spent time outside for the majority of the day.

Factory farm–raised chickens live in deplorable conditions. The corporations that run factory farms cram chickens into spaces so small they cannot sit down or flap their wings. Many of the birds get sick and die, so they are pumped full of antibiotics, a practice that results in antibiotic-resistant bacteria that are passed directly to you.

In addition to the brutal conditions in which the animals are raised, you want to avoid eating conventionally raised poultry for a number of health reasons. The ammonia and bad bacteria from the crowded, filthy conditions in which they live can contaminate the meat. Industrially raised chickens are fed low-quality feed that contains pesticides, herbicides, and fungicides as well as GMO grains. The antibiotics used to keep the chickens alive not only produce super bacteria but also mess with the gut microbiome, killing off important microbes of anyone who eats the meat. Humans also absorb the hormones the birds are fed to make them grow quickly. Some scientists say those hormones contribute to early onset puberty in children, which is becoming more common. The fear that poultry experience during slaughter elevates the levels of stress hormones—cortisol, adrenaline, and other steroids—in the meat. The chemical profile of stress is passed to consumers, increasing inflammation.

Organic chicken is a mainstay of my diet, because it has so many health benefits. Chicken provides:

* A lean source of protein, which promotes muscle growth.
* Tryptophan, which increases serotonin levels in the brain. The calming effect enhances your mood, relieves stress, and helps you attain restorative sleep. Since this amino acid is present in both chicken and turkey, poultry is a natural antidepressant.
* Phosphorus, which supports the health of your teeth and bones.
* Selenium, an essential mineral, which improves metabolic performance, including the regulation of your immune system.
* Vitamin B_6, which boosts your metabolism to burn more calories and contributes to the health of your blood vessels.
* Niacin, which guards against cancer and DNA damage.
* Vitamin A, a powerful antioxidant, which keeps your eyes healthy and fights inflammation.
* Vitamin B_6 and omega-3 fatty acid, which improve heart health by reducing inflammation in the blood vessels.

In one study, chicken soup was found to inhibit the migration of neutrophils, reducing inflammation during common infections, scientific proof that a steaming bowl of chicken soup actually has healing properties.

As you now know, free-range chicken deserves a place on my superfood list. If you find chicken boring—"Chicken again?"—just wait until you try my recipes.

FREE-RANGE EGGS: THEY'VE TAKEN A BEATING

Eggs, like red meat, cheese, and coconut oil, have been demonized by health organizations. After decades of propaganda that eating eggs is a direct path to high cholesterol levels and heart disease, eggs have won acceptance again as nature's multivitamin, the most nutritious food you can eat. The fact is that eggs and dietary cholesterol do not negatively affect cholesterol levels in the blood. Eggs will improve your cholesterol profile. Eggs raise good HDL and change bad LDL cholesterol from dangerous small, dense LDL to large, benign LDL.

Eggs contain small amounts of almost every vitamin and mineral required by the human body, including calcium, potassium, iron, zinc, manganese, Vitamin E, and folate, to name a few.

One large egg contains:

1. Vitamin B_{12}: 9% [of the RDA]
2. Vitamin B_2 (riboflavin): 15%
3. Vitamin A: 6%
4. Vitamin B_5: 7%
5. Selenium: 22%

Eggs are loaded with high-quality proteins, good fats such as omega-3s, and trace nutrients such as phosphorous, selenium, and choline, which affects the brain. Ninety percent of people in the United States are choline deficient. The body uses twenty-one amino acids to build proteins. Nine of those are essential amino acids, which have to come from what you eat. Eggs are rich in these essential building blocks. If you have been depriving yourself of delicious, rich egg yolks, you can stop ordering egg white omelets. Yolks contain almost all of the nutrients that make eggs a perfect food.

Eggs are high on the satiety index, keeping you feeling full. Consuming eggs can help you to lose weight and body fat.

Just as you want to buy free-range chicken, the same is true for eggs. The diet of caged hens is grain based, which changes the nutritional composition of the eggs they lay. Tests have found that pasture-raised hens produce eggs that are more nutritious than factory-farmed eggs. Here are some of the test results comparing free-range with factory-farmed eggs:

- ⅓ less cholesterol
- ¼ less saturated fat
- ⅔ more Vitamin A
- Two times more omega-3 fatty acids
- Three to six times more Vitamin D
- Three times more Vitamin E
- Seven times more beta-carotene

These figures demonstrate clearly that you will get more for your money if you buy organic free-range eggs.

Another beautiful thing about eggs is that they are very versatile.

GRASS-FED BEEF: THE CONTROVERSY CONTINUES

Eating beef has been taboo since the connection between the saturated fat in beef, cholesterol, and heart disease became generally accepted. Recent findings have shed new light on fats and heart disease that questions this assumption. Remember that Weston Price found that animal fats were needed to help the body absorb fat-soluble nutrients. The jury is still out on beef, which is why I suggest limiting your beef consumption to a four-ounce portion two or three times a week. Today the pendulum seems to be swinging toward the pro side. These are some current pros and cons, but new discoveries are being made every day:

Con: Eating beef can trigger an inflammatory response in those with a genetic predisposition.

Pro: The fat profile of beef is unique. Two of the fats it contains are stearic acid, a saturated fat, and oleic acid, the same fat found in olive oil. These fats improve cholesterol levels.

Con: Other saturated fats in beef, namely palmistic acid and myristic acid, can raise cholesterol levels. The myth that saturated fat in the diet is linked to heart disease has been debunked. Processed meat is a different story.

Pro: Along with Vitamins B_3 and B_6, iron, zinc, and selenium, beef contains some nutrients that are not available in plants, including B_{12}, creatine, an energy reserve in muscles and the brain found only in animal fats, and carnosine, an antioxidant that protects against degenerative process.

Con: When the drippings from grilled meat hit the fire, compounds called HCAs drift up into the meat. HCAs have been linked to cancer. Adding rosemary to your marinade reduces the formation of HCAs.

Pro: Eating meat can lift your spirits. A study in Australia compared women who ate one to two ounces of beef or lamb per day to a group that ate less than one ounce per day. The meat eaters were half as likely to have major depression or anxiety. Part of the outcome may be due to the fact that the beef and lamb in Australia are grass fed, which makes them higher in mood-protecting omega-3s.

Con: Carcinogens can form when meat is overcooked by any method. Make sure to cut away burned areas.

Pro: We evolved to be carnivores, eating plants and animals. Meat is one of the reasons we evolved to have big brains.

Con: The abundant iron in beef can raise the level of iron in the brain, which can increase the risk of developing Alzheimer's disease.

You will get more benefit from eating grass-fed beef. Conventional beef cattle are fed grains, mostly GMO corn, and do not graze. Cattle were meant to eat grass and plants. They are ruminant animals with a four-chambered stomach that has a unique microbiome to digest the tough cellulose found in the plants in their diets. The microbes in the part of the stomach called the rumen produce the enzyme cellulase, which digests cellulose. A diet of grain changes and diminishes the nutrients in the beef.

Beef cattle are shot up with growth hormone to bulk them out and antibiotics to keep them from getting diseased. All of that is passed on to you when you eat conventionally raised meats. Eating organic, grass-fed beef is worth the extra expense. Compared to factory-raised cattle, grass-fed beef has:

- Less total fat
- Two to six times more heart-healthy omega-3 fatty acids
- More linoleic acid, a fat that reduces heart disease and cancer risks
- More antioxidant vitamins, including Vitamin E

I think grass-fed beef is more flavorful than conventionally raised beef. It is unadulterated and fresher tasting.

GOJI BERRIES: SMALL BUT MIGHTY

Goji berries have been used in Chinese medicine for more than two thousand years. In alternative and complementary medicine circles, they are recognized as a high-antioxidant food with extensive benefits. Studies have found that they raise energy levels, athletic performance, the quality of sleep, concentration, mental acuity, calmness, and well-being, while they reduce fatigue and stress. This superfood is a great weapon in your fight against inflammation.

High in antioxidants, protein, and fiber, goji berries also contain important phytochemicals, including beta-carotene, zeaxanthin, lycopene, cryptoxanthin, lutein, and polysaccharides. What sets them apart from other fruits and berries is that they are a good source of eighteen amino acids, especially nine types considered essential that the body cannot make. They also have five sources of healthy fatty acids, such as alpha-linolenic acid and linoleic acid. They are chock full of zinc, iron, phosphorus, and riboflavin.

Their Vitamin A and C content fights free radical damage,

protecting the body from high levels of inflammation and building immunity. They help to control the release of sugar into the bloodstream and prevent the blood sugar roller coaster. By increasing insulin sensitivity and stabilizing blood sugar, goji berries naturally prevent diabetes and act as a remedy if you are having problems with your blood sugar levels. They are believed to detoxify the liver and are used as an ingredient in many liver cleanses.

You can incorporate dried goji berries into your diet easily. They are such a popular ingredient you can buy them in the health food section of most supermarkets. If you have trouble finding goji berries, you can order them online. Use them like raisins. Just toss dried goji berries into a salad, trail mix, or yogurt. You can add them to baked goods or sauces, or simply use them as a garnish for vegetables and desserts. You'll find ways to use goji berries in Chapter 15.

KALE: THE NUTRITIONAL POWERHOUSE

I know, you can't escape kale. It's the emperor of greens. To say it is everywhere is an understatement. The reason for this vegetable's runaway popularity is that it is one of the most nutrient-dense foods you can find. A cup of raw kale contains:

- Vitamin A from beta-carotene: 206% [of the RDA]
- Vitamin K: 684%
- Vitamin C: 134%
- Vitamin B_6: 9%
- Copper: 10%
- Potassium: 9%
- Magnesium: 6%
- Vitamin B_1: 3% or more
- Vitamin B_2: 3% or more
- Vitamin B_3: 3% or more

- Iron: 3% or more
- Phosphorus: 3% or more
- Fiber
- Protein
- Omega-3 fatty acid: alpha-linolenic acid

Kale is packed with powerful antioxidants such as polyphenols and the flavonoids quercetin and kaempferol. Another abundant antioxidant found in kale is beta-carotene, which the body turns into Vitamin A. The high content of Vitamin C—4.5 times higher than spinach—serves vital functions. For example, this water-soluble antioxidant is needed to synthesize collagen, an important structural protein in the body. Kale contains substances that have been shown to lower cholesterol. Steamed kale is 43 percent as potent as cholestyramine, a drug for lowering cholesterol. Kale is one of the best sources of Vitamin K. A cup of raw kale contains almost seven times the recommended daily amount. Sulforaphane, a substance that helps to fight the formation of cancer at a molecular level, is abundant in this mighty vegetable. I could go on and on about iron, calcium, and the inflammation-fighting omega-3s. And it's a great detox food that keeps your liver healthy. Adding kale to your diet is an easy way to increase the nutrients you need to stay healthy.

One of my favorite ways to prepare kale is to sauté or roast chopped kale in virgin coconut oil. Everyone has been making kale chips, but these are spectacular. I could eat mountains of kale prepared this way. You'll find the recipe on page 280.

MACADAMIA NUTS: AN INDULGENCE THAT DELIVERS

Macadamia nuts are so luxuriously sweet and creamy that it might be difficult to believe they are a healthy food. In the past, people avoided eating them, because they are high fat. We know now that eating fat does not necessarily make you fat. It depends on the fat you consume. Macadamia nuts are rich in monounsaturated fats that protect the heart and blood vessels.

Macadamias are an excellent source of many vitamins, minerals, phytonutrients, protein, and dietary fiber. Antioxidants such as polyphenols, amino acids, and flavones are part of the picture.

The monounsaturated fats in the nuts protect the heart by reducing cholesterol and triglyceride levels and helping to clean the arteries. The fat in macadamias stimulates weight loss. They are rich in palmitoleic acid and omega-7 fatty acids, which provide building blocks for the enzymes that control the burning of fat and suppress the appetite. Palmitoleic acid turns your body into a fat-burning machine and reduces fat storage.

Their high flavonoid content protects cells from environmental toxins and damage. Flavonoids convert to antioxidants in the body and go on search and destroy missions to obliterate free radicals. The oil from macadamia nuts contains oleic acid, which plays an important role in reducing inflammation. Powerful antioxidants in macadamia oil, such as squalene and Vitamin E, also neutralize free radicals. Consider macadamias a weapon against inflammation.

The phosphorus in macadamia nuts has a number of roles, including bone and teeth mineralization, metabolism, and the absorption and transportation of nutrients. Calcium also contributes to the formation of teeth and bones, and manganese helps the body to deposit new bone tissue. So eating macadamias is good for your teeth.

Just because macadamia nuts are good for you doesn't mean you should go overboard. One cup has 962 calories. Three nuts have 70 calories. It's a good idea to dole out a few nuts and to savor them. This is not a food you should binge on!

Here is an abbreviated look at the wealth of vitamins and minerals the nut delivers:

- Folates: 3% [of the RDA]
- Niacin: 15%
- Pantothenic acid: 15%
- Pyridoxine: 21%
- Riboflavin: 12%
- Thiamin: 100%
- Vitamin C: 2%
- Vitamin E: 1.5%
- Potassium: 8%
- Calcium: 8.5%
- Copper: 84%
- Iron: 34%
- Magnesium: 32.5%
- Manganese: 180%
- Phosphorous: 27%
- Selenium: 6.5%
- Zinc: 11%

EXTRA VIRGIN OLIVE OIL: LIQUID GOLD

Olive oil is at the core of a Mediterranean diet. People from that region have lower risks of heart disease, high blood pressure, and stroke and longer life expectancies compared to North Americans and Northern Europeans. The average American consumes a liter of olive oil per year compared to Greeks at twenty-four liters per person annually, Spaniards at fifteen liters, and Italians at thirteen liters.

Olive oil is composed primarily of monounsaturated fatty acids. A nutritional breakdown follows:

1. Saturated fat: 13.8% [of the RDA]
2. Monounsaturated fat: 73% (most of it oleic acid)
3. Omega-6: 9.7%
4. Omega-3: 0.76%

5. Vitamin E: 72%
6. Vitamin K: 75%

Go with extra virgin olive oil, which is unrefined and comes from the first pressing of the olives. Not only does it have the most delicate flavor, but EVO also has the highest level of beneficial plant nutrients from the olive. Of the extensive list of phytonutrients in EVO, the polyphenols are the most important because of their antioxidant and anti-inflammatory properties. Consuming as little as two tablespoons of EVO a day has been shown to have significant anti-inflammatory benefits.

Studies have shown that olive oil can decrease cholesterol and the ratio between LDL and HDL. The oleic acid in olive oil has been linked to lowered blood pressure. Olive oil improves the function of the lining of the blood vessels and can help prevent blood clotting that can develop into heart attacks and strokes. Since fat takes longer to digest than protein and carbs, olive oil keeps you feeling fuller longer. Monounsaturated fat enhances the breakdown of stored fat, and you know that excess fat contributes to inflammation.

The health benefits of olive oil are significant, and of course, it is delicious.

Start making your own salad dressing with extra virgin olive oil to increase your consumption of this liquid gold.

QUINOA: COMPLETE PROTEIN IN A SEED

If you are concerned about dropping rice and pasta from your diet, quinoa (keen-wha) is the answer. It has become one of the most popular health foods, because it satisfies that craving. On the Triple A Diet, you will add quinoa to your diet in the Renew stage.

Actually, quinoa is not a cereal grain. It is a seed that is prepared and eaten as a grain. Quinoa is one of the few plant foods that contain all nine essential amino acids. It is high in fiber,

B vitamins, iron, potassium, calcium, phosphorus, Vitamin E, and many antioxidants. One cup of cooked quinoa has:

- Protein: 8 grams
- Fiber: 5 grams
- Manganese: 58% [of the RDA]
- Magnesium: 30%
- Phosphorus: 28%
- Folate: 19%
- Copper: 18%
- Iron: 15%
- Zinc: 13%
- Potassium: 9%
- Vitamins B_1, B_2, B_6: over 10%

Very high in antioxidants, quinoa becomes even more so when the seeds are sprouted. Soaking quinoa overnight in water will increase the antioxidant content. Quinoa is rich in plant flavonoids, specifically quercetin and kaempferol, which have anti-inflammatory, antiviral, anticancer, and antidepressant effects. Quinoa is gluten-free and can improve metabolic health, including lowering blood sugar and triglyceride levels.

Quinoa has become popular for good reasons. It will satisfy your carb cravings while delivering a nutritional payday.

If all of this seems like too much information, I want to explain why I went into such depth on the superfoods. These foods have such amazing properties that I wanted to give you a comprehensive picture of what they can do for your health and well-being. Knowing why a recommendation is effective is a good motivator for taking advantage of the benefits. The program in the chapters that follow incorporate these foods into the weekly meal plans. The recipes take the guesswork out of how to use these highly nutritious, anti-inflammatory ingredients to make dishes that are as delicious as they are healthy. If you think healthy food is bland and boring, be ready for some tasty treats. Dr. Gerry's superfoods will win you over.

Did you know that physical inactivity is one of the most common causes of inflammation? You will be happy to learn that you do not have to commit to long workouts to get the desired results. It's all about intensity as you will soon discover. The next chapter gives you a fitness plan that will reduce inflammation with two high-intensity workouts that take no more than thirty minutes per week as well as strategies for adding movement to your life.

Chapter Nine

Moving Just Enough

There is no way you could have avoided hearing how important it is to exercise. When you look at the list of positive effects, exercise seems like a cure-all for the many physical and mental problems that plague us today. Exercise:

- lowers the risk of developing or reverses heart disease, diabetes, high blood pressure, and cancer.
- boosts immunity.
- reduces stress.
- alleviates depression and anxiety.
- improves sleep.
- builds lean muscle mass, which burns calories at a higher rate than fat.
- maintains healthy bones and joints.
- increases coordination, flexibility, and balance.
- fights inflammation.

If the right kind of exercise can do all this and more, why are so many people sedentary?

When I ask my patients about their level of activity, many say there are just not enough hours in the day to find time to work out. The fact is that you do not have to do two-hour killer workouts in the gym every day to achieve anti-inflammatory results.

What you have to aim for is adding more movement to your life and doing high-intensity strength training twice a week.

YOU'VE GOT TO MOVE

Movement and exercise are different. You need both to fight inflammation and to raise your level of fitness. I like to think of movement as recreation. Look at the roots of the word: create again. It's about restoring yourself. Movement means getting up from your chair and doing something you enjoy to renew yourself. You might take the dog for a long walk, do yoga, or ride a bike outside. I don't know many people who couldn't use a daily dose of recreation.

Watching what you eat and working out a few times a week will not make up for all the time you spend being sedentary. Even if you exercise an hour a day, you have to think about what you are doing for the other twenty-three hours. Most people spend a major portion of their time sitting—in cars, buses, or trains, at their desks or conference room tables at work, at restaurants, in front of computer screens or television. American adults spend 55 to 70 percent of their time sitting or lying on a couch. That's about eight or fifteen hours of waking time. If you add seven hours spent sleeping, your sedentary time can add up to twenty-two hours. Why is sitting too long bad for you? These reasons should persuade you to get moving:

- When you sit, the powerful muscles of your legs and butt do not contract. The electrical activity in your muscles drops. Your muscles require less fuel, which causes the amount of blood sugar in your bloodstream to rise. A high level of blood sugar contributes to inflammation and to the development of diabetes.
- The level of enzymes that break down and remove harmful fat in the bloodstream falls, which leads to an unhealthy balance between good and bad cholesterol.

- The rate at which your body burns calories drops to a third of what it would burn if you got up and walked.
- Sitting can cause your cells to die prematurely and affects your genes.
- Inactivity changes the neurons in your brain that control heart rate, blood pressure, and breathing. The changed neurons can cause blood pressure to rise and contribute to cardiovascular disease.
- One study showed that being physically active helps balance the microbiome, by encouraging beneficial microbes in the gut to thrive, decreasing the risk for inflammation. The sedentary subjects of the study had high markers for inflammation in their bloodstream.

Research has gone on to show that simply standing more is good for you. Some studies have recommended that you get up every twenty minutes and stand for two minutes or walk twenty feet. There are anti–sitting apps, such as Time Out or Break Reminder, that will notify you when it is time to get up. You don't have to buy a treadmill desk. You don't have to push yourself with a demanding regimen you know you will never keep up. You just have to build more movement into your life. Making small adjustments to your daily routine will get you going.

TEN EASY WAYS TO MOVE MORE

You are surrounded by energy-saving devices. My question is, why are you saving energy? Energy you do not burn turns to fat, and an excess of fat leads to inflammation. The more energy you burn, the more energy you'll have. You will tap into a deep reservoir of energy you didn't know was there. Aside from significant health benefits, you will feel so much better once you start moving more.

I could give you an endless list of small ways to make movement a part of your life. These suggestions are only a beginning. My intent is to get you thinking about all the little things you can do to be more active that are not a big deal.

1. Take a walk after each meal.
2. If you take a subway, bus, or train to work, stand for part of your commute.
3. Get off public transportation a stop earlier or park farther away and walk to where you are going.
4. Play music and dance when you do housework.
5. Get up for water every odd or even hour. Not only will you be moving, but you will also be well hydrated.
6. At the end of your workday, clear off your desk and stand when you do it.
7. When you talk on the phone, stand or pace.
8. Hide your remote controls.
9. Don't carry your cell phone with you at home. Get up to answer it when it rings. Same with landlines.
10. Don't stagnate or head for the kitchen during TV commercials. Do a chore, stretch, or work out your arms with resistance bands.

You get the idea. When you think about how "convenience" is rendering you sedentary, you will find so many ways to step up your activity. Make simple physical activity a habit, and you'll discover renewed energy that will change your life. Now that you're moving, it's time to take it to the next level.

WHY EXERCISE IS AN EFFECTIVE DE-STRESSOR

One important way exercise helps to improve your health is that it can turn off your body's reaction to stress. When you encounter a physical threat, the primitive fight-or-flight response kicks in to give you energy to escape or confront that threat. Though you are not likely to be charged by an angry rhino in the parking lot of the grocery store, emotional, social, or work stress evokes the same acute response. The problem is that psychological stress does not get resolved quickly and does not need the increased energy it generates. The inflammatory cascade produced by the stress response, which involves more than fifteen hundred bio-chemical reactions, becomes chronically activated. By-products of the stress response, such as cortisol, continue to circulate in your body, causing inflammation.

By using the energy produced by stress, exercise removes the potentially damaging by-products of the fight-or-flight response and allows the body to return to balance. To put it more simply, since the physical stress response prepares the body for physical action, physical activity is a natural way to prevent harmful con-sequences by completing the process. Exercise can turn off that inflammatory cascade.

EVERYONE CAN FIND THIRTY MINUTES A WEEK TO EXERCISE

With the help of my friend Adam Zickerman, owner of InForm Fitness and author of the *New York Times* bestseller *Power of 10*, we are going to give you two high-intensity strength-training programs that take no more than fifteen minutes twice a week. No excuses. Anyone can find fifteen minutes two days a week to squeeze in a safe and efficient muscle-building routine that can be done anywhere. The only equipment you will need is resistance bands, which are easy enough to take with you wherever you go—even the office.

ON RESISTANCE BANDS

Resistance bands are inexpensive and easy to buy online or in stores. It's a good idea to buy a set of bands, because as you get stronger, you will progress to a band with higher resistance.

You can buy bands that are simply a long piece of rubber. A set comes in different lengths and levels of resistance. You can wrap or double up bands without handles for greater control of the resistance level.

The other type of resistance equipment is a set of tube resistance bands. These bands are made of rubber or cord of different lengths. I recommend getting a set with foam or plastic handles. Foam handles are superior, because they cushion your hands and protect them against soreness or blisters. Foam handles will give you a firmer grip as well. Some sets have cuffs for different workouts. The workout in this chapter is designed to be done with simple bands or tubes with handles—it's up to you. Be certain the bands or tubes you use are made of high-quality material. You do not want them to snap as you work out with intensity.

HIGH INTENSITY IS THE WAY TO GO

Adam Zickerman, a pioneer in the super-slow, high-intensity movement, has designed two strength and conditioning programs to help you fight inflammation. I have asked him to explain high-intensity exercise and describe the workout in his own words. Over to Adam:

The essence of the training in my gyms and the workout in this book centers around slowing the pace of weight training and focusing on fatiguing every muscle. That means repeating an exercise to muscle failure. You only have to do this fifteen-minute routine twice a week. Most of us spend fifteen minutes just coming up with excuses to avoid exercising. Combined with proper nutrition and rest, the high-intensity, muscle-building workout I have designed will give you the power to fight inflammation and to reshape your body safely and effectively, regardless of your age, physical condition, or lifestyle. As I have witnessed again and again, you will have better results with this anti-inflammatory workout than with other, more time-consuming fitness routines.

Long-term strength and health depend on building and maintaining as much muscle as possible. The best way to build muscle is to work with light to moderate resistance very slowly. Each time you do an exercise, count ten seconds up and ten seconds down. Move in a very controlled way. One rep equals twenty seconds. Keep the tension of the move in your muscle, not the joint. Once you have completed the move, do it again without resting, and again, until you can no longer move the muscles you are working. They burn, you shake, and finally you are in muscle failure. The slow movement works to build muscle without any harmful side effects or risks normally associated with high-intensity workouts. You will not experience wear and tear on your joints, ligaments, and other connective tissue.

I repeat: Muscles have to be worked to the point of failure if you want to see results. By failure, I mean working a muscle group to the point at which you have no more force left to give— not even an ounce, no matter how hard you push. This can be very uncomfortable. I call it "hitting the wall." You are fighting the resistance, unable to move another inch. Once you pass the point of muscle exhaustion, cross the threshold and continue trying to lift to a count of ten, even though you have hit the wall. You will not be able to make the band move. That final ten seconds of straining after you pass the point of failure is when the payoff happens.

If you push yourself to that level, you will collect the real prize. For the short term, you have earned a break for three or four days. If you exercise to muscle exhaustion, you must allow time for the muscles to rest and repair so that your body can respond and begin to build muscle. You should only do this workout twice a week. After each workout, you must rest your muscles for three or four days for proper muscle recovery. Microtears in muscle fibers need time to repair, which is how muscle is built. Trying to overdo these workouts is actually counterproductive. You will end up breaking down muscle tissue. If you follow the plan long term, you will safely maintain a level of fitness and release proteins that fight inflammation

It is critical to understand the level of intensity required for results. Most people stop short. They feel discomfort and think they are hurting themselves. When new clients start training with me, they are often ready to stop when they are at 80 percent of muscle failure. So don't stop your reps too soon. Keep pushing until you can't do more reps.

During each exercise, use deep inhalations to push up and release the breath as you come down. Proper breathing super-oxygenates your muscles and produces the most efficient workout.

WHY HIGH-INTENSITY EXERCISE FIGHTS INFLAMMATION

For years, intense exercise was considered a cause of inflammation. When you "feel the burn," you have pushed your muscles to a new level. High-intensity exercise makes a muscle work hard, producing minute tears, and forces your body to repair and build new muscle tissue. The natural response to intense exercise is inflammation. When muscles contract, the body also releases myokines, a type of cytokine, which increases insulin sensitivity and glucose use inside the cells of your muscles. Myokines also promote the release of fat from cells in fat tissue and the burning of fat in the muscle. These myokines end up helping to control chronic inflammation by inhibiting the release and effect of inflammatory cytokines, which fat produces.

When a muscle contracts, it releases the myokine interleukin-6 (IL-6). When IL-6 is released from a muscle in high concentrations, it stimulates an anti-inflammatory cascade in which inflammatory inhibitors, including anti-inflammatory cytokine IL-10, are produced.

High-intensity resistance training releases signaling molecules that trigger a healing response that uses inflammatory and anti-inflammatory reactions to repair and strengthen muscle tissue. High-intensity, short-duration movement is the most efficient way to fight inflammation with exercise.

THE MIND⇔BODY CONNECTION HIGH-INTENSITY STRENGTH TRAINING

Adam has designed two full-body programs of six exercises each. The beauty of these workouts is that you can make them as challenging as you want by choosing the amount of resistance the bands offer. If you are using graduated bands or cords, it's time to move up to the next level of resistance when it takes more than fifteen minutes to complete the series. When muscle failure takes longer, you are getting stronger. If you are not challenging your muscles, you will reduce the benefits of the exercise.

I've prepared two workouts—primarily because it's good to change it up now and then. One is not more difficult than the other. When the routine you are doing becomes boring, try the other one. You can go back and forth as often as you want, because both high-intensity routines work all the major muscle groups in your body.

There are hundreds of moves you can perform with your resistance bands. When you are ready to create your own workout, you can find countless exercises, arranged by muscle groups, online.

Make doing these routines twice a week a habit. It should be automatic, like brushing your teeth. My patients tell me that doing high-intensity resistance training on Tuesday or Wednesday and one during the weekend works well for them. When you work out is up to you, but be certain to allow your muscles to rest between workouts.

CHALLENGE 1

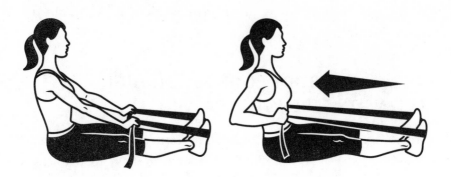

EXERCISE 1: SEATED ROW

Target: Back
- Erector spinae in the lower back
- Middle and lower trapezius in the upper back
- Rhomboids and latissimus dorsi in the middle back
- Teres major in the outer back

For maximum benefit and to avoid injuring your back, be certain to sit up straight with your shoulders squared while doing this exercise.

1. Sit on the floor with your legs extended in front of you. Wrap the resistance band or cord securely under your feet. Hold the band at a point that allows you to sit up straight.
2. Pull the band to each side of your torso with your elbows bent close to your sides until your shoulder blades squeeze together.
3. Pause in this position and then return to start with your back remaining straight.
4. Repeat until muscle failure and you cannot do another one.

EXERCISE 2: STANDING SHOULDER PRESS

Target: Shoulders and arms

- Anterior, medial, and posterior deltoids
- Biceps
- Triceps

1. Step on the center of the band with your feet shoulder-width apart. Hold the handle or the end of the band in each hand, bending your elbows and bringing your upper arms slightly lower than your shoulders with your wrists directly above your elbows.

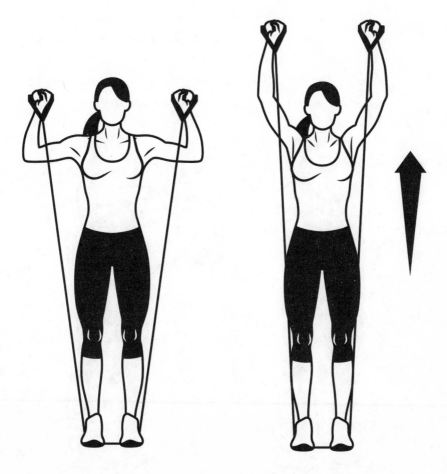

2. With your palms facing forward, raise your arms above your head until they are straight.
3. Lower your arms slowly.
4. Repeat the exercise until muscle failure.

EXERCISE 3: CHEST PRESS

Target: Front of chest and arms
  * Pectoralis major
  * Anterior deltoids
  * Triceps

1. You can anchor your band in a door if you have a set with an anchor or wrap it around a weight-bearing pole, such as a metal stair rail. The safest way to do this exercise is to place the band behind your back at chest height and to wrap any excess length around your forearms.

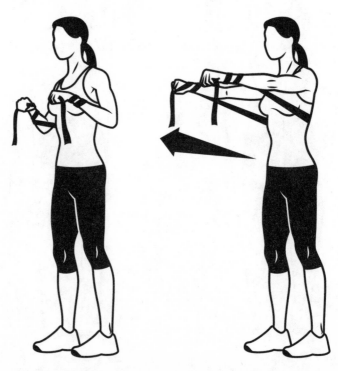

2. With elbows at your sides and your arms at a 90-degree angle, push straight out. Be sure to keep your shoulders down.

3. Resist the band as you return to your starting position.

4. Repeat the movement until muscle exhaustion and you cannot do more reps.

Exercise 4: Kickbacks

Target: Butt

- Gluteus maximus
- Hamstring

1. Place the resistance band around your right foot and get down in all-fours position.

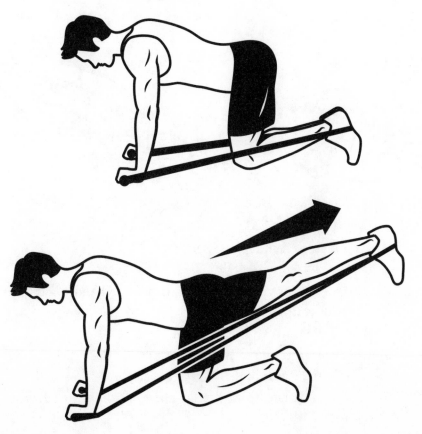

2. Kick back and up with your right foot and straighten your leg.
3. Resisting the band, slowly lower your right leg and bring your knee to the floor in starting position.
4. Repeat until muscle failure.
5. Put the resistance band on your left foot and repeat the exercise until you can no longer do it.

EXERCISE 5: LEG PRESS

Target: Quadriceps

- Gluteus maximus
- Hamstrings

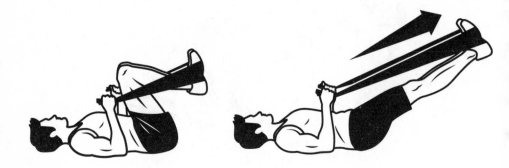

Bands not crossed and legs lower.

1. Sit on a mat or carpeted area and lace the band under the arches of your feet.
2. Roll down until your back is flat.
3. Hold the band by the handles or increase the resistance by holding the bands higher with less slack.
4. Bend your knees toward your chest and hold in tabletop position.

5. Press through your feet to straighten your legs. Avoid arching your back by pulling your belly button into your spine.
6. While keeping your abs tight, bend your knees back into starting position.
7. Repeat the movement to muscle exhaustion.

EXERCISE 6: TORSO TWIST

Target: Core
- Abs
- Obliques

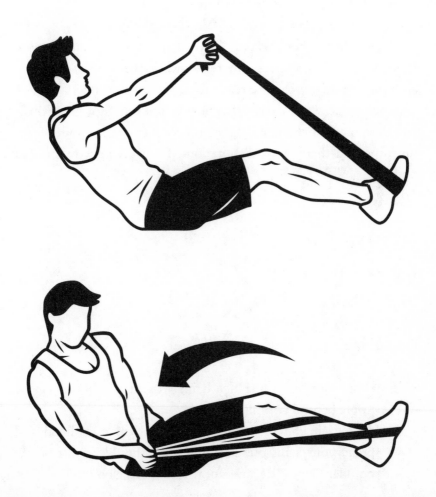

1. Sit on the floor with your knees bent and your feet flat on the floor.
2. Wrap the resistance band around your feet and grab the handles or band together with both hands.
3. Lean back so that your torso is at a 45-degree angle to the floor. Make sure your spine is flat and not rounded.
4. Put your arms out in front of you with one hand on top of the other.
5. Slowly rotate to the right as far as you can, trying to tap the floor.
6. Rotate to the left, tap the floor, and rotate to the right.
7. Continue until muscle failure.

Remember, when it takes more than fifteen minutes to do these six exercises, increase the resistance of the band or cord you are using. Your muscles are ready for a bigger challenge.

The second set of exercises is below. They are not more difficult than the first challenge. Since it's good to change your workout now and then to avoid boredom, I am giving you another option.

CHALLENGE 2

Exercise 1: Fly

Target: Chest
- Pectoralis major
- Deltoids

1. Either loop the resistance band around a stable object or simply behind your back.
2. Hold each end of the resistance band in each hand and spread your arms out straight. They should be just below shoulder height. Be sure not to lock your elbows.

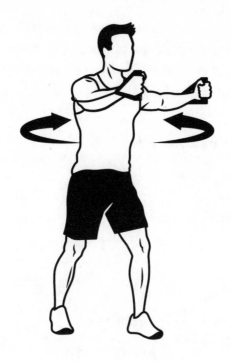

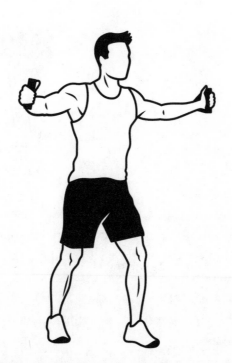

3. Inhale as you bring both arms forward until your hands meet in front of your chest. Keep your elbows slightly bent.
4. Exhale as you return to the starting position.
5. Repeat until muscle failure.

EXERCISE 2: PULL-APARTS

Target: Shoulders and middle back
- Shoulders
- Middle back
- Traps

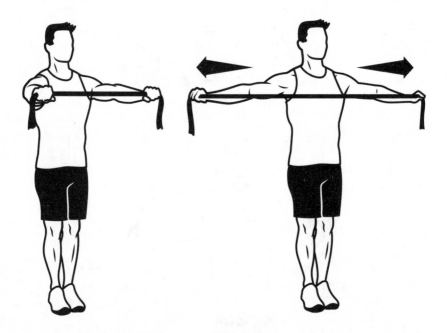

You can modify the difficulty of this exercise by changing the amount of slack you have in the band before you open your arms. More slack will make the exercise easier, and a tighter band will offer more resistance.

1. Stand with your feet shoulder-width apart and a light bend in your knees.

2. Hold the exercise band in front of you with your hands slightly lower than your shoulders. Keep your elbows slightly soft to avoid hyperextension.

3. As you exhale, pull your abs to your spine to stabilize your torso as you open your arms to the side. Avoid arching your back and pushing your rib cage forward. Concentrate on your shoulder blades sliding together.

4. Inhale as you slowly return your arms to starting position.

5. Repeat to muscle failure.

EXERCISE 3: SQUAT

Target: Lower back and legs

- Erectorspinae
- Gluteus maximus
- Quadriceps
- Hamstrings

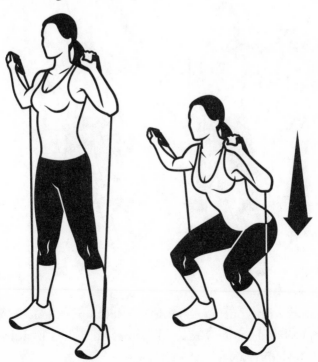

1. Hold the handles of the band in both hands and step onto it with your feet shoulder-width apart.
2. With your palms facing you, bring your hands up to your shoulders.
3. Bend your knees and squat down slowly as if you are going to sit. Your butt drops back as you lower. Keep your knees pointed forward and over your toes.
4. Return slowly to standing and repeat until muscle failure.

EXERCISE 4: SIDE BENDS

Target: Sides of your waist or love handles

- Obliques

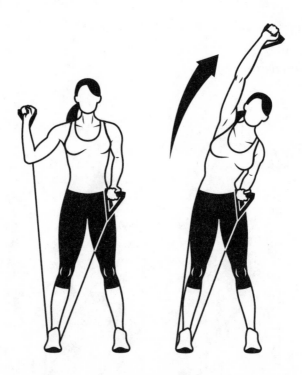

1. Stand with your feet shoulder-width apart. Place the resistance band under your right foot and hold a handle or end of the band in each hand.

2. Place your left hand at hip level with your fist facing up. Your right hand should be shoulder height with your elbow bent, palm forward.

3. Press the right hand overhead. Reach and bend to the left.

4. Keeping your core tight, return to your upright starting position.

5. Repeat the movement to muscle failure.

6. Repeat the exercise with the band under your left foot, your right hand at your waist, and your left hand at shoulder height.

7. Reach up with your left hand and bend to the right.

8. Repeat to muscle failure.

EXERCISE 5: LYING STRAIGHT LEG RAISES

Target: Hips and lower abdomen
- Hip flexors
- Abs

1. Lie on your back and wrap the middle of the band around both feet.

2. Hold the ends of the resistance bands in each hand.

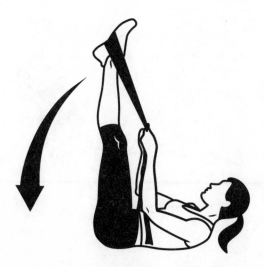

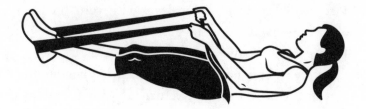

3. Raise your legs a little less than 90 degrees in the air. Make sure you do not arch your back while doing this exercise. Your tailbone should be heavy.
4. Slowly lower your legs until your feet are a few inches from the ground.
5. Then raise your legs with control to the starting position.
6. Repeat until muscle failure.

EXERCISE 6: GLUTE BRIDGE

Target: Butt
- Glutes
- Abs
- Erector spinae
- Hamstrings
- Adductors

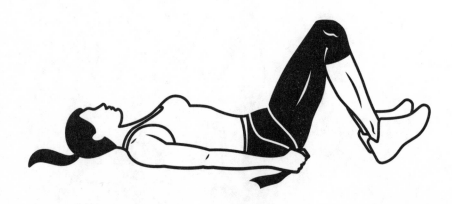

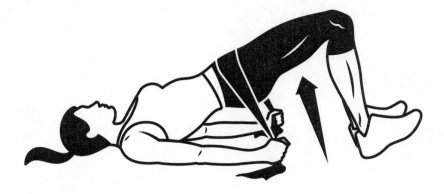

1. Lie on your back with your knees bent and your feet flexed, hip-width apart.
2. Place the band across your pelvis. Hold it taut and press the ends of the band into the floor beside the hips.
3. Pull your abs in tightly, squeeze your glutes, and push your hips up into a bridge.
4. Hold for 1 count and then slowly lower for three counts to starting position.
5. Repeat until muscle failure.

So far in Part 2, you have learned three aspects of the Cura-tola Care Program: groundbreaking information on protecting your mouth's microbiome, the way to eat to curb oral and systemic inflammation, and efficient movement and high-intensity exercise techniques that will turn off the stress-induced, highly inflammatory fight-or-flight response. The next chapter will give you relaxation techniques to counter stress.

Chapter Ten

Calm Counts

If your life is a juggling act, and your "to do" list is overwhelming, you are not alone. The demands of modern living are only intensifying. There is a lot of noise out there. Not only are you on call twenty-four/seven, available to receive texts, e-mails, and phone calls, but you are also checking Twitter and responding to Facebook, LinkedIn, and other social media outlets. The electronic universe is just one focus of your attention. You seem to live in a state of constant stress. You might have young children to raise, rebellious teenagers to protect, a demanding job, aging parents to care for. Maybe your credit cards are maxed out or you face a six-figure debt in college loans. You've been on what seems like hundreds of job interviews and can't seem to land one. Or your company is downsizing, and you don't know where you stand. You don't have to be in crisis mode, such as going through a divorce, getting fired, or losing a loved one, to feel stressed out. You can find yourself close to road rage when you are stuck in daily traffic jams. Long lines make you grind your teeth. Neighbors' playing loud music or office politics can wind you up. Nothing is static in our society. The strain of adapting to and coping with a changing environment is what life is all about. Science has found that the cumulative effects of everyday situations can have a profound impact on your health and feelings of well-being. Stress is an inflammation trigger.

If you live in a state of chronic psychological stress, as most of us do, your body loses its ability to control inflammatory responses. Stress enhances inflammation, an important immune response. As you know, inflammation is an overactive cytokine response, which leads to physical deterioration from your gums to your brain. Not getting enough restorative sleep, one of the plagues of modern life, also increases the level of pro-inflammatory cytokines. When feeling under tremendous pressure for the long term, you are more susceptible to the development and progression to a wide range of diseases, from the common cold to cancer.

Remember the fight-or-flight response I described in the last chapter? The hormone cortisol is the main culprit in the stress-illness connection. When your brain senses danger, the hormones epinephrine, also known as adrenaline, and norepinephrine join cortisol to increase heart rate and respiration and the availability of glucose so that you are ready to run away or fight. Cortisol shuts or slows down other processes in the body that use up energy, including digestion, reproduction, physical growth, and immune function. The brain does not distinguish between a physical threat and psychological distress. The perception of a threat can trigger this hormonal cascade. **If you experience negative emotions such as anger as your default mode, your body is in a constant state of fight or flight.**

Current research has found that chronic stress can bias the brain to perceive more danger by changing the regions that govern the perception and response to a threat. Prolonged exposure to cortisol inhibits the growth of new neurons in the brain and can cause increased growth of the portion of the brain that controls emotional responses, including fear. When this happens, your expectation of threats in the environment is heightened, and you see threats everywhere.

Stress hormones also repress neuron growth in the brain area that contributes to forming new memories. Stress impairs your memory and diminishes your brain's ability to put emotional memories in context. To put it simply, experiencing too much stress makes you forget not to be stressed out. This is a vicious cycle: The stress hormones cause you to perceive more threat, and your body reacts with an increased stress response.

Psychology affects biology in another important way. The effects of stress play out in the way genes express themselves in the immune system. Chronic stress changes the gene activity of immune cells before they enter the bloodstream. The immune cells are primed to fight infection or trauma, even when there is no infection to fight, which results in increased inflammation. The chronic inflammation that results is a long-term, runaway activation of the immune system's defense response.

You can break this destructive cycle by learning to calm your mind and body. This part of the Curatola Care Program adds a mental and spiritual component to the cleansing, nutritional, and exercise fundamentals. Including mindfulness meditation and anti-inflammatory yoga positions in your routine will support everything else you are doing to redirect your trajectory from decline to vibrant health.

MINDFULNESS MEDITATION

The thought of meditation might bring to mind a yogi sitting in a cave turning inward for days on end. You do not have to go to extremes to benefit from mindfulness meditation. In the broadest terms, meditation reduces stress, and consequently inflammation and the risk of disease that goes along with the chronic condition. Meditation produces measurable health benefits throughout the body.

Research has found that meditating can change the shape, volume, and connectivity of your brain. **Several studies have shown that meditating promotes more communication**

among parts of the brain that process stress-related reactions and other regions related to focus and calm. Meditation enhances the connection between two areas of the brain that typically work in opposition. The first region is called the default mode network, involved in mind wandering, daydreaming, and internal reflection. The other region is the executive attention network that regulates focus, planning, and decision making. When the brain's circuits are rewired by meditation, the improved executive control results in stress resilience. The overall effect is that your brain becomes more able to manage stress.

These brain changes contribute to reducing inflammation as well. One study found lower levels of the pro-inflammatory biomarker, IL-6, in subjects who meditated as compared to those who simply practiced relaxation techniques. Epigenetic research has discovered that meditation can reduce the expression of genes that drive the process of inflammation.

Many believe that meditation involves blocking out your thoughts and having a blank mind. Nothing could be further from the truth. **Mindfulness meditation involves focusing your awareness in the present moment.** While you meditate, you focus your attention on your breath, bodily sensations, and the thoughts that come to your mind without being judgmental. You simply acknowledge emotions and thoughts as they arise without reacting to them. Your aim is to experience an open, receptive, nonjudgmental awareness of the present moment.

BEING IN THE MOMENT—HOW TO GET THERE

It is so easy to waste emotional energy regretting the past and worrying about the future, or missing the past and expecting a better future. The purpose of meditating is to ground yourself in the present exactly as it is. You might find starting your meditation practice challenging, but stay with it. You will find yourself becoming more open to your experiences, even difficult ones, and will be less likely to overreact even when you are not meditating. Changes are going on in your brain that will decrease the intensity of your reaction to stress.

To begin, you have to commit to finding time to meditate every day, starting with five minutes. It is best to meditate in the morning and the evening. You might want to start with five minutes only once a day. The Curatola Care Program lengthens your meditation time each week.

Preparation

Pick a place that will allow you to sit without interruptions. Set your phone or a kitchen timer so that you are not distracted by wondering when your session will be over. Sit in a comfortable chair with your feet on the floor or on a cushion with your legs crossed in front of you.

Be aware of your posture. Sit erect with your shoulders back. You should feel as if your spine is elongated, being pulled from the top of your head. Don't force it or be stiff. You should be relaxed, your spine stable and strong. Keep your elbows by your sides and place your hands and forearms on your thighs. You are ready to train your mind.

The Practice

1. Settle into your chair and meditating posture. If you find yourself nodding off or getting hazy as you meditate, check your posture, which should keep you relaxed but awake.
2. Close your eyes, or focus your open eyes downward, out a couple of inches from your nose.
3. Focus on your five senses. Experience the sounds, scents, tactile feelings, taste, and vision of the moment. Feel your hands resting on your thighs—the texture of your clothing

or the warmth of your skin. Hear the hum of the air conditioner. Smell the flowers in the vase next to you. Taste the mint that was in your iced tea. Observe the colors floating behind your closed eyelids. This will ground you in the present.

4. Remaining in the moment you have created with your senses, turn your attention to the flow of your breath as you inhale and exhale. This focus on your breath will contrast to what is going on in your mind. Your breath will keep you anchored to the present moment.

5. Let your breath move naturally in and out. You might want to strengthen your focus by thinking "in" as you inhale and "out" as you exhale. With each breath, you become more relaxed.

6. Inevitably thoughts will come to mind. You might think about what you are going to have for dinner, be irritated by something your partner said the previous night, or worry about whether you are going to make the deadline for a project in the office.

7. When you notice what is happening, return your attention to your breath. Just let the thought go. Don't judge yourself or what you are feeling or thinking. Some find it helpful to label the thought "thinking" in their minds as they turn their focus to their breath.

8. You go away, and you come back to the here and now. Shifting your awareness from thought to the experience of the present moment is the practice of meditation.

That's all there is to it. Mindfulness meditation is simple, yet powerful. Sitting and doing nothing can help you achieve peace of mind and harmony as well as reduce systemic inflammation. The time you set aside for meditation could be the most productive five minutes of your day.

SUBDUING INFLAMMATION WITH YOGA

Yoga has been practiced for thousands of years. Many consider it an ancient science. For those of you who consider yoga a throwback to "New Age" hippy times, scientists are proving that assumption wrong. A study at Ohio State looked at two hundred breast cancer survivors who had never practiced yoga. Half the group continued not practicing yoga, while the other half took ninety-minute classes twice a week for twelve weeks and took home DVDs. The group that practiced yoga reported less fatigue and higher energy levels than the other half of the group three months later. Blood tests before and after the experiment measured three inflammatory cytokines in the bloodstream. After three months of yoga, the three markers for inflammation in the yoga group were lower by 10 to 15 percent. Other studies that measured biological markers found that expert yoga practitioners had lower inflammatory response to stress than beginners.

I have selected seven deeply relaxing positions that will restore you and balance your mind, body, and spirit. These calming postures can help reduce pain in the joints and can quiet the fight-or-flight response. The practice of restorative yoga can reduce inflammation, lower blood pressure, slow your heart rate, and calm your nervous system. Assuming any one of these poses and holding it for a designated amount of time while breathing deeply will melt tension and stress away. If you feel pain in any of your joints as you do a posture, stop immediately and try another one that is more comfortable.

As you are doing these poses, enjoy how your body feels and focus on living in your body rather than your mind. This will go a long way to temper inflammation caused by our mind's reaction to stress.

When you concentrate hard, you tend to tighten your facial expression as well as your hands. Be conscious of softening your face and hands, because relaxing these areas will send feedback to the mind to relax.

SEVEN ANTI-INFLAMMATORY YOGA POSES FOR DEEP RELAXATION

Equipment

As with meditating, I recommend you have a quiet, pleasant space in which you can practice without interruption. You might want to invest in some yoga equipment, namely:

* A yoga mat
* Two blocks
* A bolster
* A blanket or two

Before buying the equipment, you can substitute blankets, pillows, and towels.

Breath

How you breathe is always an important element of yoga. As you do in meditation, you will focus on your breath, but you will do deep breathing while doing yoga. With your mouth closed, pull air in deeply. Let your stomach expand on the inhale. Exhale slowly through the nostrils. This deep breathing will calm your body and refresh you. In fact, breathing this way whenever you are stressed is like having a natural tranquilizer at your disposal. It's a technique you can use anyplace, anytime.

Child's Pose

This is one of my favorite postures. It targets the muscles in the buttocks and lower back, which is great for those of you who spend a lot of time sitting in front of a computer all day.

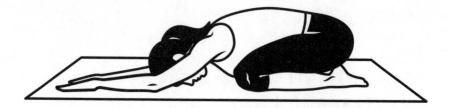

- Position yourself toward the back of your mat. Get on your knees and drop your buttocks to your heels.
- If you feel tension in your knees, you can slip a folded blanket between your buttocks and calves as a cushion and support.
- Bend forward from your hips until your chest rests on your knees.
- Rest your forehead on the floor. If your range of movement is limited, you can rest your head on your fists or use a block.
- Reach forward with your arms with your palms flat on the floor. Rest for two to five minutes.
- To get out of position, lift your head and walk your hands back to your sides. Come to an upright seated position.

Reclining Bowed Angel Pose

The posture targets your hips and thighs, especially the inner groin.

- Place a bolster or folded blanket lengthwise on your mat.
- Start to recline by lowering onto your elbows and then lying on the bolster. Position the bolster under your rib cage and a folded blanket under your head to support your neck.
- Place your arms on either side of your body, palms up.

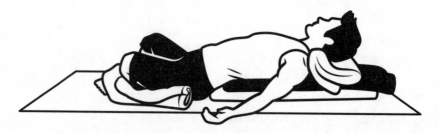

- Bring the soles of your feet together and let your knees fall to the side.
- Place a block or a pillow under each thigh for support.
- Close your eyes, breathe deeply, and relax.
- Rest for three to five minutes.

Happy Baby Pose

This posture is great for opening up the hips, stretching the hamstrings, and releasing the lower back.

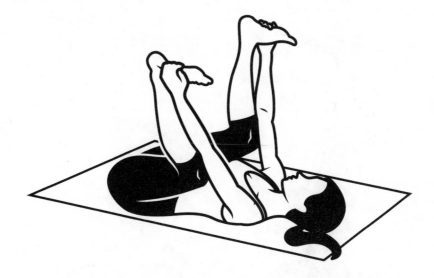

- Lie faceup on your mat.
- Draw your knees to your chest with your arms.
- Grab the outside of each knee with a hand and draw your knees open and down.
- Relax your lower back.
- For a deeper stretch, grab the sole of your right foot with your right hand and your left foot with your left hand.
- Draw your feet down so that knees come toward the floor on each side. Be sure to keep your ankles over your knees.

- Hold for one minute as you breathe deeply. Make sure your spine is flat on the floor.
- Then return your feet to the mat.
- You can repeat if you would like.

Fountain of Youth or Legs Up the Wall Pose

If you want the stress of the day to melt away, try this cooling posture. It eases muscle tension and lower back pain, lowers blood pressure, and relieves stress and fatigue.

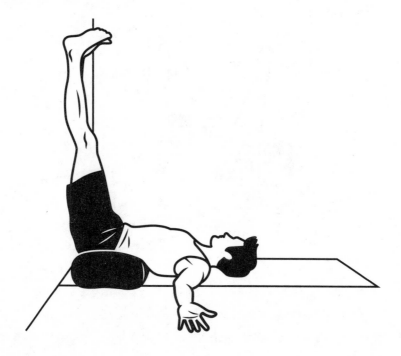

- Move your mat perpendicular to the wall. Roll up a towel or have your bolster close by.
- Lie on your back and raise your legs so that they are resting against the wall.
- Push your feet against the wall and lift your hips.
- Place the bolster or rolled towel under your pelvis.

- Relax your pelvis down to the bolster and rest your legs against the wall again.
- Keep your back flat.
- Extend your arms to the side in a comfortable position, palms up.
- Relax in that position, breathing deeply, for five minutes.
- To get out of the position, let your knees tuck to your chest, then roll slowly to your right side. Use your left hand to push yourself to a seated position.

Warrior II

This pose increases flexibility in the hips and shoulders and increases strength in the legs, back, and ankles.

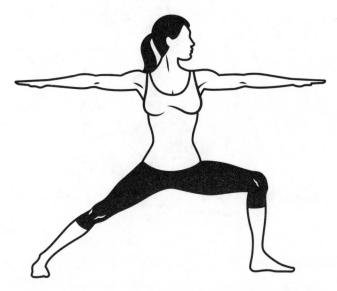

- Position your feet about three to five feet apart.
- Press down through your feet to bring your torso erect as you align your shoulders above your hips.
- Turn your right foot forward and your left foot parallel to the back of the mat, pointing slightly inward so that your hips and shoulders are facing your torso.

- Bend your right knee over your ankle and stretch your arms apart, right arm in front of you, left arm in back as you look over your right hand.
- Hold for thirty seconds and build to a minute.
- Repeat on your other side.

Lord of the Fish Pose or Seated Spinal Twist

This posture massages the internal organs and rejuvenates the spine. It's excellent for the digestive system.

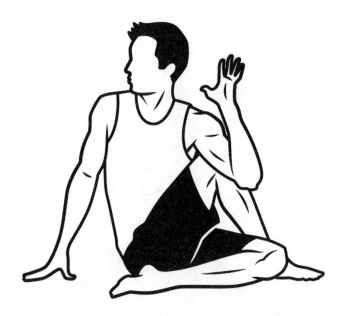

- If you need lower back support and help tilting your pelvis forward, sit on the folded edge of a blanket.
- Extend your left leg.
- Sitting tall, bend your right knee and place your right foot next to the left knee.
- Place your right hand on the floor behind your body with your fingers pointing behind you.
- Hook the left elbow to the inside of the right knee.

- As you inhale, lift and lengthen your spine.
- Exhale and twist your spine so that you are looking over your right shoulder.
- Hold the position for five deep breaths.
- Repeat on the other side.

Seated Eagle Pose

This posture loosens tension in the neck and shoulders that can produce headaches. You can sit on the floor with crossed legs or in a chair.

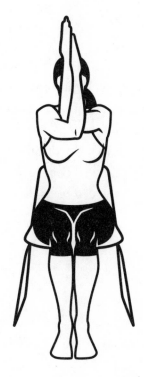

- Cross your right arm over your left and touch the backs of your palms together. If you are unable to get into that position, put your palms together.
- Drop your head toward your arms.

- Breathe deeply through your upper back.
- Close your eyes and relax for a minute.
- Repeat with your left arm over your right.

You might enjoy doing five minutes of yoga at the end of the day. Experiment with these seven postures. Notice where tension is trapped in your body and choose a position that will relax that area. You can do one posture at a time or do a series. It's up to you.

With the stress busters in this chapter, you have what you need to begin the program and change your life.

You now have the knowledge you need to reclaim your vitality, robust health, and *joie de vivre*. Part 3 presents the 28-Day Cura-tola Care Program: Rethink, Restore, Renew, and Refresh. I will map out what you need to do in each stage and provide you with a schedule to show you how easy it is to incorporate changes into your life. There are a month's worth of meal plans and over sixty easy-to-prepare recipes that will convince you that eating to keep your microbiome in balance can be as delicious as it is healthy.

PART III

THE 28-DAY CURATOLA CARE PROGRAM

Chapter Eleven

Week 1

Rethink/Clean Up

You have made the decision to take control of your health. Congratulations! You will soon be on your way to achieving the renewed energy and radiance that result from cooling down the inflammation that is incrementally sapping your strength and destroying your body down to the cellular level.

Your commitment is the most important aspect of your makeover. Determination is all you need for my plan to work for you. If you follow the program for twenty-eight days, you will see and feel improvements that will encourage you to make these fundamental changes a routine part of your life for the long term. As I mentioned earlier in the book, consult with your doctor before beginning this program.

My 28-Day Program will make it easy to do away with those things in your life that are ruining your health and to replace them with practices that will promote your sense of well-being. Just a month on the program will make you feel better than ever. My goal in this part of the book is to walk you step-by-step through the adjustments you will be making in each week of the program. You will be making four lifestyle changes:

- Nutrition
- Healthy exercise
- Stress reduction

- Supplementation in the form of vitamins, minerals, enzymes, amino acids, and botanicals

You learned what you need to do to clean up your act in Part 2 of the book. During the first week on the program, you have to identify the habits that are hurting you. The first phase of the program is to rethink the choices that you make every day. As I've said before, I like to call it "getting the junk out of the trunk." For the first week of the plan, you have to assess how toxic you are and how to lower your toxic load.

DETOX TO CLEAR THE WAY

There are a few simple things you can do to kick off your new campaign. This is a list of some of the actions to take before you begin the program.

For oral hygiene:

1. See your dentist to discover what condition your teeth and gums are in.
2. Schedule a cleaning or periodontal treatment if necessary.
3. Discuss with your dentist a plan to replace failing "silver" (amalgam) fillings with a safe removal protocol.
4. Replace your toothbrushes with new soft brushes. Get an electric or battery-operated toothbrush if you think using one will inspire you to brush longer.
5. Get rid of toothpaste and mouthwash that will destroy the balance of your oral microbiome. Either make homemade substitutes or select products from the list on page 85.
6. Make sure you have floss and/or interdental flossing brushes on hand. Try to floss twice a day—before brushing your teeth in the morning and before bed. I promise, making this a habit will greatly improve your oral health.

Reducing toxic exposure:

1. Study the labels of your personal grooming products. Chances are, most of them are filled with toxins. Check out the Environmental Working Group's website: www.EWG .org. They have a database called Skin Deep that rates skin care, nail, hair, sunscreens, fragrance, shaving, and baby care products.

2. The Environmental Working Group also has a "Guide to Healthy Cleaning," in which they rate 2,500 products, including all-purpose, laundry, kitchen floor, bathroom, dishwasher, and furniture products. It's a valuable resource. You might not want to toss everything out immediately, but as you use up products, think about replacing them with others that are less toxic.

Revising what you eat:

1. Get rid of all the junk food—chips, pretzels, cookies, cake, candy, crackers, ice cream. They only feed your inflammation.

2. Remove all processed food from your kitchen—from the refrigerator, freezer, and pantry. That includes frozen entrées and snacks, most canned foods (organic beans are the exception), and salad dressings. Read the labels. If there are ingredients that you can't pronounce on the label, the product is on the toss-out list.

3. Get rid of fruit juices, sports drinks, and sodas, including diet.

4. Put away hard liquor for guests and forget the wine and beer, at least for the twenty-eight days of the program.

5. There is no place in your kitchen for anything white, with the exception of cauliflower and organic dairy products. Say good-bye to bread, rolls, biscuits, pasta, and white rice.

The Clean Fifteen and the Dirty Dozen

Organic vegetables cost about a third more than conventionally grown produce. If this is a problem for your budget, the Environmental Working Group has an annual list of foods that are clean, called The Clean Fifteen. You do not have to buy organic produce for fruits and vegetables on this list. They also rate The Dirty Dozen, foods that test high in toxins that you should try to buy organic. They put out new lists annually.

When referring to the "Clean" list, remember that you will not be eating a lot of fruit the first week, because so many fruits are high in sugar.

To check these lists, go to the Environmental Working Group website at www.EWG.org.

These lists are good guides if you want to include some conventionally grown produce when you shop. Of course, locally grown produce, even if not organic, is better for you than industrially produced vegetables and fruits that are shipped long distance.

Remember that the Environmental Working Group puts out new lists each year, and they do change.

Restock your kitchen with:

1. Bottled or filtered water. You might want to have a water filter pitcher or faucet.
2. Take a look at the recipes for lacto-fermented food beginning on page 234 and get hold of the salt, whey, or starter culture you will need to make this important part of your diet.
3. Make sure you have free-range, organic eggs.
4. Always have avocados on hand.

5. Give extra virgin olive oil and coconut oil a front and center place on your shelves.

6. Stock your freezer with individually wrapped organic boneless chicken breasts and a whole chicken for roasting.

7. Take the time to sprout some nuts and seeds—almonds, walnuts, macadamia nuts, and pumpkin seeds are a great snack. See page 109 for sprouting directions.

8. Get some dried goji berries to add to salads and trail mix.

9. Have organic vegetables for crudités on hand: carrots, celery, cherry tomatoes, cucumbers, broccoli, cauliflower, snow pea pods.

10. Stock up on kale, which you can turn into chips with some extra virgin coconut oil. (See recipe, page 280.)

11. Make bone broth and freeze it. You will be able to sip on it all day. (See recipe, page 246.)

12. Purchase some pint and quart mason jars for making lacto-fermented vegetables. Since the fermentation process takes time, look over the recipes that begin on page 234 and try a recipe or two right away so that the vegetables will be ready when you start the program or shortly after you do.

13. Study the meal plans on pages 192–223 and purchase a few days' worth of ingredients in advance.

Food Focus for Rethink/Clean Up

Make a radical break from your old habits and start new with clean food that will set you on the path to reducing inflammation. During this week, you are doing a chemical detox by avoiding foods filled with preservatives, dyes, bad fats, excess salt, and sugar by cutting out processed foods. You are eliminating detrimental foods and your toxin backlog. Your shift from fast

food and sugars focuses on what I call "getting the white out."
These are your food goals for the first week of the program:

- Replace one meal a day with a Super Smile Smoothie or a
  protein smoothie of your choice.
- Add lacto-fermented foods.
- No processed foods.
- No fruit.
- No grains.
- No bread, pasta.
- No cookies, candy, sweetened drinks.

SUPPLEMENTS

You will be taking supplements the first week of the program
to counter the withdrawal you may experience from dropping
sugar and simple carbohydrates from your diet. The supplement
plan this week is designed to quiet any cravings you might have
for the foods you have sworn off. Since your aim is to rid your
body of toxins, I've worked in supplements that will support the
detoxification process. Again, be sure to check with your physi-
cians before adding supplements to your regimen.

The supplements incorporated during the Rethink phase of
the program focus on providing support for the elimination of
sugars and toxins, while preparing the body for transformation
and restoration.

You will be taking four supplements each day. On page 191,
you will find a side bar that shows you what a day during Week 1
looks like.

These are the supplements for the Rethink phase of the program:

Synulin: A natural blend of chromium and botanical ingredients for glucose metabolism and physical sugar withdrawal symptoms. This is a terrific nutritional product that includes 1mg of a
unique patented chromium (Chromium 4-hydroxyisoleucinate),

which assists in improving glucose metabolism and reducing insulin resistance.

Take 1 capsule twice per day at mealtime.

Neurosyn: A natural blend of Vitamins B_1 and B_6, amino acids, and botanicals to support neurological enhancement for neurotransmitter metabolism. Neurosyn balances acetylcholine, serotonin, and dopamine for focus and cognitive support while helping to minimize the psychological effects of sugar withdrawal "blues."

Take 1 capsule twice a day in the morning and lunch with or without meals.

Spectra One: The first 100 percent certified organic, completely plant-based, full-spectrum multivitamin/multimineral supplement. Rich in natural B vitamins, the Vitamin B_{12} (hydroxocobalamin) in Spectra One is synthesized by bacteria, just as probiotics do in the human GI tract, which maximizes absorption. This supplement is a cellular healing formula that improves the body's ability to absorb and digest food properly while eliminating waste and toxins. Spectra One provides a broad array of water-soluble nutrients.

Take 1 capsule twice per day with or without meals.

Spectra Two: The other half of the complete Spectra "duo," Spectra Two delivers a comprehensive supply of the fat-soluble vitamins including beta-carotene (Vitamin A), borage (GLA), coenzyme Q10, sea buckthorn, tocotrienols/tocopherols, Vitamin D_3, and Vitamin K_2. Together, Spectra One and Spectra Two provide a unique combination of cellular food for optimal bioavailability of vitamins, minerals, and fats.

Take 1 dropper twice per day with Spectra One between meals.

EXERCISE EQUIPMENT

You no doubt already have clothing and comfortable shoes for recreation and workouts. You will need to have simple exercise bands or bands with handles for the High-Intensity Workout, which you will begin in Week 2.

JUST DIVE IN

To make the changes you want to occur quickly, you have to go cold turkey on sugar and simple carbs. Since most food addictions involve simple carbs—also known as "comfort" food—giving them up can be challenging. As you'll see from the meal plans, the food you will be eating is delicious and abundant. It's about making the right choices. Though the changes in your diet this first week are radical, your body needs shaking up, and you will feel the results after a few days. Instead of thinking about unhealthy snacks and meals, you can shift your attention to the physical and mental activity you will be adding to your day.

BUILDING IN TIME FOR EXERCISE AND RELAXATION

This first week you will ease into the other aspects of the program and build over the twenty-eight days. Making exercise, meditation, and relaxation techniques a habit will boost your mood and energy as they fight inflammation.

MEDITATION (5 MINUTES DAILY)

Most people with a meditation practice start their day by meditating. Calming your mind down can make you more resilient and less affected by the ups and downs of the day to come. If you choose to meditate in the morning, I suggest you do so before you exercise or have breakfast. Meditating soon after eating is not recommended.

Some people prefer to meditate later in the day to manage the stress that has built up. You should experiment and decide which is best for you.

RECREATION/MOVEMENT (10 MINUTES)

It's time to stop being a couch potato. If you want to stay healthy, you have to move more. Adam Zickerman likes to think of this sort of movement as recreation. Whether it's walking, taking a bike ride or a Zumba class, gardening, even standing at your desk every twenty minutes, or playing with children, you need to up your level of activity.

If you are mostly sedentary, then start with just ten minutes of walking. Taking a walk after a meal is a good routine to adopt. As you advance in the program and you are at peak energy, you will find yourself craving movement.

RELAXATION POSTURES (5 MINUTES DAILY)

The seven yoga postures found on pages 173–180 will de-stress you and fight inflammation. You can do them all in a sequence or any number you want. You might like to pick one that targets an area in which you feel tension to begin, and then add other postures as needed. These can be done before you meditate or in the evening before you go to bed. Ridding your body of tension at the end of the day can help you get a good night's sleep. If you are experiencing a stress SOS, you can always do a relaxation posture in your office or cubicle or take some time wherever you are.

A Day on Week 1: Rethink/Clean Up

Meditation: 5 minutes*
Breakfast: protein smoothie of your choice (see recipes, pages 230–233)
Supplements with breakfast: 1 capsule Synulin, 1 capsule Neurosyn

Snack

Supplements without meals: 1 capsule Spectra One, 1 dropper
Spectra Two

Lunch

Supplement with lunch: 1 capsule Neurosyn

Movement/recreation: 10 minutes

Dinner

Supplement with dinner: 1 capsule Synulin

Relaxation postures before bed, but no sooner than 40 minutes
after dinner: 5 minutes†

Supplements without food: 1 capsule Spectra One, 1 dropper
Spectra Two

*Depending on what you prefer, you can meditate before dinner rather
than in the morning.
†Relaxation techniques can be done before dinner or following workouts
as well.

You have to play with the schedule to see what works best for you. People tend to have a natural biorhythm to their day, but then you never know what a day will serve up. An extremely demanding day might require a different balance. Be sensitive to your ups and downs and plan your program schedule accordingly to stay on an even keel.

At the start, I suggest you follow the same schedule every day. If you start switching it up before these practices become automatic, it's easy to skip one and never manage to fit it into your busy day. Being too fluid can undercut your progress. Stick with a schedule if you want to see and feel improvements.

MEAL PLANS FOR WEEK 1

In creating the meal plans, I took into account how busy you probably are. I tried to build leftovers into the program and include food you can make ahead. If you are like most of my patients, you tend to eat habitually. If you have trail mix on hand, you eat it as a snack until you've finished it. These meal plans are very varied. They are suggestions about the way you can eat on the Triple A Diet. You have to tailor them to work for you. Though I aimed to give you easy-to-make dishes, if you find that a meal requires too much preparation, switch it out for a simpler day or a simpler version of a dish. (See Chapter 15 for the complete recipes.)

Prepare in advance to save time during the week:

Bone Broth (page 246)
Grace's Blast-Off Bars (page 280)
Peak Energy Trail Mix (page 282)
Hard-boiled eggs
Cauliflower Rice (page 272)

It helps to have tasty snacks on hand when you are going cold turkey on simple carbs.

If you haven't already, it is also a good idea to get working on some lacto-fermented vegetables (recipes on pages 234–239). If you don't have a jump start on preparing lacto-fermented vegetables, you may have to incorporate them later.

Day 1

Breakfast
    Protein smoothie of your choice (recipe suggestions pages
        230–233)

Midmorning snack
    Celery with almond butter

Lunch
    Spinach salad with mushrooms, bacon, hard-boiled egg, and
        avocado

Afternoon snack
    Peak Energy Trail Mix (recipe page 282)

Dinner
> Roasted whole chicken or store-bought rotisserie chicken
> Crispy Roasted Vegetables—carrots, Brussels sprouts, broccoli,
> parsnips—whatever appeals to you (recipe page 279)

Day 2

Breakfast
> Protein smoothie of your choice

Midmorning Snack
> 8 ounces of Greek yogurt with chopped walnuts

Lunch
> Mixed green salad with cold chicken leftovers and goat cheese

Snack
> Leftover roasted veggies

Dinner
> Cajun Blackened Arctic Char (recipe page 260)
> Spaghetti squash with pesto sauce
> Old-Fashioned Dill Pickled Green Beans (recipe page 235—
> though this has to be made in advance)

Day 3

Breakfast
> Protein smoothie of your choice

Midmorning Snack
> Bone Broth (recipe page 246)

Lunch
> Sliced tomatoes, mozzarella, and fresh basil drizzled with olive oil

Snack
> Guacamole with crudités

Dinner
> Broiled or grilled steak
> I Can't Believe It's Not Mashed Potatoes (recipe page 269)
> Steamed asparagus with a grated hard-boiled egg on top

Day 4

Breakfast
Protein smoothie of your choice

Midmorning snack
2 hard-boiled eggs

Lunch
Superfood Special: Kale, Avocado, and Olive Salad (recipe page 277)

Snack
Peak Energy Trail Mix (recipe page 282)

Dinner
Boil and peel shrimp in Old Bay Seasoning
Roasted Brussels sprouts

Day 5

Breakfast
Protein smoothie of your choice

Midmorning Snack
Macadamia nuts

Lunch
Hamburger, chicken, turkey, or veggie burger with cheddar or Swiss cheese, onion, lettuce, avocado slices, and pickled asparagus

Snack
Bone Broth (recipe page 246)

Dinner
Broiled Country Mustard Chicken (recipe page 255)
Cauliflower Fried Rice (recipe page 273)

Day 6

Breakfast
Protein smoothie of your choice

Midmorning Snack
Peak Energy Trail Mix (recipe page 282)

Lunch
Lettuce roll-up
Think of the lettuce as bread or a wrap and fill with slices of fresh
roast beef, turkey, ham, or cheese, lettuce, any of the
lacto-fermented vegetables, salsa.

Snack
Mixed olives with extra virgin olive oil and red pepper flakes

Dinner
Guilt-Free Pizza of your choice (see recipe pages 262–264)

Day 7

Breakfast
Protein smoothie of your choice

Midmorning snack
Grace's Blast-Off Bar (see recipe page 280)

Lunch
Bone Broth (recipe page 246)
Salsa with a Kick (see recipe page 234) and crudités

Snack
Tropical Kale Chips (recipe page 280)

Dinner
Meatless or Meaty Chili (see recipe page 261)
Tropical Kale Chips (recipe page 280) or Cauliflower Fried Rice
(see page 273)

Chapter Twelve

Weeks 2 and 3

Restore/Shift the Balance

The aim of this stage is to shift the balance from inflamed to healing. You have already begun to reduce inflammation in a dramatic way by eliminating the toxins and the sugar from your diet on the first week of the program. At this stage, your body will be working hard as it begins to return to equilibrium and to repair any damage that inflammation has caused. The Triple A Diet will speed the process.

Food Focus for Weeks 2 and 3: Restore/Shift the Balance

You began to rid your body of the buildup of toxic chemicals during Week 1. Your aim in the second and third weeks of the Curatola Care Program is to lay the foundation for restoring your health. This can be achieved by:

- Restoring balance and biodiversity of the oral and gut microbiome and body processes.
- Building a foundation and routine that shift dietary habits to healthy choices.

- Using supplements to raise the level of glutathione protection in the body, resolve inflammation, and provide probiotic and prebiotic support.
- Controlling protein portions.
- Eating more alkaline and antioxidant rich foods.
- Incorporating more of Dr. Gerry's superfoods (see Chapter 8).

The Restore stage of the program will demonstrate that eating an anti-inflammatory diet is not about deprivation. You'll be adding a wide variety of foods that support your transition to health.

PORTION SMARTS

You know that eating supersized portions makes no sense, but it's easy to go over the top and have that king–size steak, work your way through an entire bowl of nuts, or pour on the salad dressing.

I don't expect you to have measuring cups and spoons handy whenever you eat, but you should be able to eyeball a portion and estimate how much is there. The following comparison of serving sizes to everyday objects should help.

Serving Size	Same As
1 teaspoon	Tip of your thumb
1 tablespoon	Poker chip
1 ounce or 2 tablespoons	Ping-Pong ball
¼ cup	One egg
½ cup	Computer mouse
¾ cup	Tennis ball
1 cup	Baseball
3 ounces of fish	Checkbook
4 ounces of fish	Two eggs
3 ounces of chicken or meat	Deck of cards
4 ounces of chicken or meat	Two eggs

CURATOLA RECOMMENDED PORTIONS

To help you take the guesswork out of it, this list will give you an idea of appropriate portions on foods that are easy to supersize unintentionally:

Homemade salad dressings	1 to 2 tablespoons
Raw almonds	12 nuts
Raw walnuts	4 to 8 halves
Raw cashews	10 nuts
Raw macadamia nuts	10 nuts
Raw pistachios	10 to 20 nuts
Sunflower or pumpkin seeds	½ ounce
Nut butters	1 tablespoon
Cheese	1 ounce (two dice)
Guacamole	2 to 3 tablespoons
Hummus	2 to 4 tablespoons
Cooked quinoa (Week 4)	½ cup as side dish, 1 cup as main course

GO TO ALKALINE FOODS

The good news is that you can eat an unlimited quantity of most vegetables, which are alkaline. Forget the white potatoes, though! Incorporating more of these vegetables along with legumes, sprouts, and nuts into your diet will go a long way to bringing your body back into balance. Though this information appeared earlier in a different format, I have repeated it here because it is so important for you to know the foods that will help you achieve balance.

Vegetables

Asparagus

Basil

Beets

Broccoli

Brussels sprouts

Cabbage

Carrot

Cauliflower

Celery

Chard

Chili

Chives

Collards

Coriander

Cucumber

Dandelion

Endive

Garlic

Green beans

Kale

Kelp

Lettuce

Onion

Parsley

Peas

Pepper

Pumpkin

Radish

Snow peas

Spinach

Sweet potato

Watercress

Zucchini

Legumes

Chickpeas

Lentils

Lima beans

Mung beans

Navy beans

Red beans

White beans

Sprouts

Alfalfa sprouts

Amaranth sprouts

Broccoli sprouts

Kamut sprouts

Mung bean sprouts

Quinoa sprouts

Spelt sprouts

For this stage of the program, stay away from fruits.

The supplements introduced in the Restore phase help to raise the body's antioxidant protection, healthy cholesterol function, healthy immune function, and prebiotic and probiotic support for digestive health while boosting support for the regulation and resolution of chronic inflammation, detoxification, cellular healing, and weight loss. At Week 2, you will stop taking Synulin and Neurosyn, but hold on to those supplements. If you fall off the wagon, you will go back on a detox regimen.

The new supplements you will be taking are the following:

GCEL: A unique natural blend of botanicals and acetyl-glutathione designed to help boost the body's production of glutathione peroxidase, a primary antioxidant throughout the body. Acetyl-glutathione is better able to avoid degradation in the digestive tract. Glutathione plays an important role in protecting the body against oxidative stress and detoxifying harmful compounds.

Take 1 capsule twice a day with breakfast and dinner.

MBC (Microbiome Colonizer): A very high potency, ten species, enteric-coated, probiotic formula designed to recolonize the gastrointestinal tract microbiome with beneficial, high attachment species. These probiotics support a healthy immune function, healthy digestion, and processing of nascent vitamins, which support the brain and cellular metabolic processes.

Take 2 to 4 capsules daily with meals.

RPM (Resolvents, Protectants, and Maresins): A blend of omega-3 essential fatty acids, which are fat-based compounds called pro-resolvents, pro-protectants, and pro-maresins. These fatty acids help mediate the body's immune function in relation to resolving chronic inflammation.

Take 2 to 4 gel capsules daily with meals.

FBR (Fibers for Intestinal Health): A blend of insoluble and soluble prebiotic fibers, herbs, whole food organic sprouts, and probiotics that support healthy cardiovascular, colon, and bowel function while assisting with healthy digestion and elimination of toxins. Sprouted seeds provide nourishment and fiber to support normal blood sugar levels. I like that this is also a psyllium-free product.

Take 1 to 2 scoops of powder per day in a smoothie, other liquids, or foods.

HIGH-INTENSITY RESISTANCE WORKOUT (UP TO 15 MINUTES TWICE A WEEK)

Now that you are moving more, you will add the high-intensity workout to your routine. I do not mean that you have to go to a gym and exercise for two hours to build muscle. Muscle-building exercise on the Curatola Care Program takes up to fifteen minutes twice a week.

Most of my patients prefer to do one session midweek and the other on the weekend. The beauty of these workouts is that the stronger you get, the longer it will take you to complete the routine, but a workout is never more than fifteen minutes long. When your workout begins to take more than fifteen minutes, you have to increase the resistance of the bands. You can change the resistance by moving your hands on the band, wrapping the cord or band around your wrist, or standing on the band to shorten it. That way you can make the exercises more difficult without changing the workout and keep your exercise time to fifteen minutes.

You can do these workouts anywhere—even behind a closed office door. And you can pack the bands wherever you go.

A total of thirty minutes a week to build healthy muscles is not much to ask. Think about how often you spend fifteen minutes randomly surfing the Internet or checking Facebook. Remember: These exercises are designed to reshape your body by creating lean muscle mass, which actually burns more calories.

When you exercise is up to you. Exercising in the morning can raise your metabolism for the rest of the day and help you to hit the ground running. If you're not a morning person and stumble from bed straight to the activities of the day, you might enjoy exercising after work or before the kids come home from school. Forget that glass of wine—get moving! Your increased energy will make you fresh and ready for the evening.

MEDITATION (WEEK 2: 7MINUTES; WEEK 3: UP TO 10 MINUTES)

I hope you are already experiencing the benefits of taking a little time to yourself to unwind. If you have, you shouldn't have a problem devoting a little more time each day to releasing tension in your mind and body.

RECREATION/MOVEMENT (WEEK 2: 15 MINUTES; WEEK 3: 20 MINUTES)

During this two-week stage of the program, you will increase the amount of everyday activity in your life. You can achieve this so easily. Don't use the remote control on your TV. Get up to change stations instead. Have a leisurely stroll after dinner or window shop at lunchtime. Meet a friend for a walk instead of sitting down for a cup of coffee. Get off the bus a stop before your destination and walk the difference. You get the idea.

RELAXATION POSTURES (FROM 5 TO 10 MINUTES)

You can do a single posture or any number of combinations. It all depends on where you feel tension trapped in your body.

A Day on Weeks 2 and 3: Restore

Meditation (Week 2: 7 minutes; Week 3: 10 minutes)*
Breakfast: You do not have to stick to a protein smoothie. You can add eggs and eat a bigger breakfast as you will see in the meal plans. (See menu plans beginning on page 204)
Supplements with breakfast:
1 capsule GCEL

2 to 4 capsules MBC

2 to 4 capsules RPM

1 to 2 scoops FBR

Snack

Supplements without food:

1 capsule Spectra One

1 dropper Spectra Two

Lunch

Movement/Recreation (Week 2: 15 minutes; Week 3: 20 minutes)

Dinner

Supplement with dinner:

1 capsule GCEL

Relaxation postures at least 40 minutes after dinner or before
   bed (5–10 minutes)†

Supplements without food:

1 capsule Spectra One

1 dropper Spectra Two

*Depending on what you prefer, you can meditate before dinner rather
than in the morning.
†Relaxation techniques can be done before dinner or following workouts
as well.

MENU PLANS FOR WEEKS 2 AND 3

During Week 2, you do not need to have a smoothie for breakfast
every day, but if it works for you, keep it up. It is important to
start your day with protein, because it will keep you feeling full
longer and help you to avoid the blood sugar roller coaster.

The make-ahead recipes for Week 2:

Goji Almond Butter Truffles (see recipe page 283)

Frittata Cupcake of your choice (see recipe page 241)

Basic Chia Cereal (see recipe page 240)

Healing Chicken Soup (see recipe page 248) or Chicken Zoodle Detox Soup (see recipe page 249)
Cauliflower Rice (see recipe page 272)

You should have plenty of Grace's Blast-Off Bars, Peak Energy
Trail Mix, and Bone Broth left. If not, take the time to refresh
your supply.

WEEK 2

Day 1

Breakfast
2 Frittata Cupcakes (see recipe pages 241–244)

Midmorning snack
Raw almonds

Lunch
Healing Chicken Soup (see recipe page 248)
Tossed green salad with sunflower seeds for crunch

Snack
Goji Almond Butter Truffles (recipe page 283)

Dinner
Coconut Chicken Breasts (page 252)
Cucumber and Celery Refresher (recipe page 277)

Day 2

Breakfast
Protein smoothie of your choice

Midmorning snack
Grace's Blast-Off Bar (recipe page 280)

Lunch
Cobb salad of roast turkey, bacon, avocado, Swiss cheese

Snack

Peak Energy Trail Mix (recipe page 282)

Dinner

Meatless or Meaty Chili (see recipe page 261) over Cauliflower Fried Rice (see page 273) served with avocado slices, grated cheese of choice, and a dollop of sour cream

Day 3

Breakfast

Fried eggs topped with chili and avocado slices

Midmorning snack

Bone Broth (recipe page 246)

Lunch

Lettuce roll-up with fillings of choice

Snack

1 Frittata Cupcake (recipe pages 241–244)

Dinner

Turkey or beef meatloaf
Centerpiece Cauliflower (see recipe page 270)
Fermented or steamed green beans

Day 4

Breakfast

Basic Chia Cereal (see recipe page 240)

Midmorning snack

Bone Broth (recipe page 246)

Lunch

Turkey, chicken, or veggie burger with guacamole and salsa

Snack

Grace's Blast-Off Bar (recipe page 280)

Dinner

Georgia's Pistachio-Crusted Arctic Char with Steamed Broccoli (see recipe page 257)

Day 5

Breakfast
2 Frittata Cupcakes (recipe pages 241–244)

Midmorning snack
Greek yogurt with cacao and sliced almonds

Lunch
Cold sliced meatloaf leftovers with lacto-fermented vegetables

Snack
Mixed nuts

Dinner
Healing Chicken Soup (recipe page 248) or Chicken Zoodle
Detox Soup (recipe page 249) with Crispy Roasted Vegetables
(recipe page 279)

Day 6

Breakfast
Protein smoothie of your choice

Midmorning snack
Peak Energy Trail Mix (recipe page 282)

Lunch
Chef salad with sliced turkey, ham, cheese of choice, olives

Snack
Grace's Blast-Off Bar (recipe page 280)

Dinner
Lemon Chicken with Sliced Almonds (see recipe page 251)
Brown Butter Drizzled Cauliflower Steaks (see recipe page 268)

Day 7

Breakfast
2 eggs any style with 2 slices of bacon

Midmorning snack
Goji Almond Butter Truffles (recipe page 283)

Lunch
　　Curried Chicken Salad in Lettuce Packages (see recipe page 254)

Snack
　　Goji Almond Butter Truffles (see recipe page 283)

Dinner
　　Boil and peel shrimp in Old Bay Seasoning
　　Roasted veggies of choice

WEEK 3

You should be getting the idea by now. A little planning will give you so many appealing choices of healthy things to eat. At this point, you should be able to satisfy your cravings with food from the Triple A Diet.

To cut down on cooking during the week, you could make some of the food for the week in advance.

The make-ahead recipes for Week 3:

Chia Goji Berry Breakfast Pudding (see recipe page 241)
Coconut Bliss Balls (see recipe page 283)
Tropical Kale Chips (see recipe page 280)
Meatless or Meaty Chili (see recipe page 261)
Cauliflower Rice (see recipe page 272)

Check on your supply of Frittata Cupcakes, Bone Broth, and Grace's Blast-Off Bars.

Day 1

Breakfast
　　2 Frittata Cupcakes (recipe pages 241–244)

Snack
　　Tropical Kale Chips (recipe page 280)

Lunch

    Cobb salad of sliced or cubed turkey, bacon, avocado, grated Swiss
      cheese, and hard-boiled egg

Snack

    Peak Energy Trail Mix (recipe page 282)

Dinner

    Stir-fried chicken and broccoli on a bed of Cauliflower
      Rice (recipe page 272)

Day 2

Breakfast

    Protein smoothie of your choice

Midmorning snack

    Hard-boiled egg

Lunch

    Healing Chicken Soup (recipe page 248) and salad

Snack

    Marinated artichoke hearts or one of the lacto-fermented veggies

Dinner

    Meatless or Meaty Chili (recipe page 261) on Cauliflower Rice
      (recipe page 272)

Day 3

Breakfast

    Chia Goji Berry Breakfast Pudding (recipe page 241)

Midmorning snack

    Grace's Blast-Off Bar (recipe page 280)

Lunch

    Leftover chili

Snack

    Coconut Bliss Balls (recipe page 283)

Dinner

Let the Good Times Roll Spicy Pecan Chicken (see recipe page 255)

Mediterranean Oven–Roasted Cauliflower (see recipe page 267)

Day 4

Breakfast

2 Frittata Cupcakes (recipe pages 241–244)

Midmorning snack

Yogurt with cocoa and sliced almonds

Lunch

Slices of leftover Let the Good Times Roll Spicy Pecan Chicken (recipe page 255) on a bed of spinach (raw or steamed)

Snack

Celery with almond butter

Dinner

Baked Arctic Char with a Scallion Crust (see recipe page 258)

Sautéed carrot rounds with herbs of choice

String beans with sliced almonds

Day 5

Breakfast

Southwestern omelet with onions, peppers, and tomatoes or Salsa with a Kick (recipe page 234) with 2 slices of bacon

Midmorning snack

Grace's Blast-Off Bar (recipe page 280)

Lunch

Build your own roll-up

Snack

Peak Energy Trail Mix (recipe page 282)

Dinner

Beef, turkey, chicken, or veggie burger with avocado slices, Tangy Grape Tomatoes (see recipe page 236), and Cauliflower Fried Rice (see recipe page 273)

Day 6

Breakfast
Chia Goji Berry Breakfast Pudding (recipe page 241)

Midmorning Snack
Mixed nuts

Lunch
Superfood Special: Kale, Avocado, and Olive Salad (recipe page 277)

Snack
1 Frittata Cupcake (recipe pages 241–244)

Dinner
Guilt-Free Pizza of your choice (see recipe pages 262–264)

Day 7

Breakfast
Cheese scrambled eggs with two links of turkey sausage

Snack
Peak Energy Trail Mix (recipe page 282)

Lunch
Build your own roll-up

Snack
Tropical Kale Chips (recipe page 280)

Dinner
Grilled or broiled steak with Mediterranean Oven-Roasted
Cauliflower (see recipe page 267) and a tossed salad

Chapter Thirteen

Week 4 and After

Renew/The New Lifestyle

As the benefits from my program begin to kick in, you probably will be hooked and want to keep the improvements going. In three weeks' time, you are moving more, using tools for relaxation, and eating a diet that is jet fuel for your body. You are in the process of renewing your body and your determination to be as healthy as you can be. Week 4 of the program is about cementing the changes you have experienced and committing to living this way for the rest of your life. In some programs, this stage is called maintenance—boring! Your goal is to do more than maintain. I want you to keep improving. This stage is designed to help you:

- Build upon the balance and diversity of the oral and gut microbiome.
- Strengthen the foundation of a new nutritional lifestyle.
- Maintain supplements that keep the body protected from inflammation, oxidative stress, and environmental toxins.

At this stage, your food choices expand and you up your movement and the amount of time you spend to regroup. Judging from my patients, taking care of yourself by following the program creates a positive energy that will improve your efficiency and productivity. Rather than dealing with the highs and lows of an energy roller coaster, you will enjoy sustained energy and an upbeat attitude. You will meet the demands of your life with renewed confidence and clarity.

Food Focus Week 4 and Beyond: Renew/The New Lifestyle

It is not realistic to expect to follow a highly restrictive diet forever. At this point, you can include some carbohydrates in your daily meals. You have to make the right choices to avoid backsliding. From Week 4 onward, you can add these foods to your diet:

* Two servings of low-sugar, high-fiber fruit
* Sweet potatoes
* Up to two portions (½ cup as a side dish) of whole grains per day

If you are creative, and the recipe section will give you some ideas, these additions will satisfy your cravings for sweets and simple carbs. I have added another energy bar, Yummy Oat Bars (page 281), which have oats in the recipe. Since oats are a grain, you cannot eat them until your fourth week.

FIGHT THOSE FREE RADICALS NATURALLY

Adding fruits to your diet is an opportunity to increase your intake of natural antioxidants, an important part of the Triple A Diet. The USDA tested one hundred foods to find those with the highest antioxidant content. There is something to be said for the phrase "eat the rainbow." Foods high in antioxidants tend to be very colorful as you will see in the list below. Most of the foods on the top twenty list are fruits. Not only will these fruits satisfy your sweet tooth, but they also help fight inflammation. These are the top twenty antioxidant foods:

1. Small red beans
2. Wild blueberries
3. Red kidney beans
4. Pinto beans
5. Cultivated blueberries
6. Cranberries
7. Artichokes
8. Blackberries
9. Prunes
10. Raspberries
11. Strawberries
12. Red delicious apples
13. Granny Smith apples
14. Pecans
15. Sweet cherries
16. Black plums
17. Black beans
18. Plums
19. Gala apples
20. Dark leafy greens

If you are mindful in your food choices, you can enjoy delicious meals and snacks as you support your body's balance in the fight against inflammation.

The New Pasta

Whole grains are a versatile addition to your diet—you can treat them as you would rice or pasta. All you have to do is add herbs and veggies to make a delicious side dish or main course. You can toss ½ cup in soup or mix the grain into a salad for texture. Grains are a rich source of protein. Quinoa, one of my superfoods, contains all the essential amino acids. Grains contain phytochemicals, antioxidants, B vitamins, Vitamin E, magnesium, iron, and fiber. Studies have shown that grains can reduce the risk of heart disease, stroke, cancer, diabetes, and obesity.

If you soak grains overnight, they become more easily digestible and their nutrients more accessible. Even better, overnight soaking reduces cooking time by ten to fifteen minutes. When you are cooking the superfood quinoa, rinse it for one or two minutes in a fine strainer before cooking, because its natural coating can be bitter.

To cook any grain:

1. Place grains and water in a saucepan.
2. Add about ½ teaspoon sea salt.
3. Cover the pot and bring to a boil over high heat.
4. Reduce the heat to low and steam for cooking time.
5. Test grain for tenderness.
6. If it needs more time and all the water has been absorbed, add ¼ cup water and cook for 5 to 10 minutes more.

The table below will give you an idea of how long it will take to prepare the most common grains. I suggest making more than you will eat in one sitting and keeping what remains in a well-sealed container in the refrigerator. Cold grains are great in a salad, mixed with cooked veggies, or as a prepared side dish that can be eaten cold.

Grain, 1 cup	Water, Cups	Cook Time, Minutes	Yield, Cups
Amaranth	2½	20-25	2½
Barley, pearled	3	50-60	3½
Buckwheat groats	2	15	2½
Millet, hulled	3-4	20-25	3½
Oat groats	3	30-40	3½
Quinoa	1¾	15-20	2¾
Rice, brown	2½	45-55	3

Grain, 1 cup	Water, Cups	Cook Time, Minutes	Yield, Cups
Rice, wild	3	50-60	4
Spelt	3-4	40-50	2½
Teff	3	5-20	3½
Triticale	3	105	2½
Wheat, bulgur	2	15	2½

Experiment with different grains. When in doubt, make quinoa, a superfood.

SUPPLEMENTS FOR WEEK 4 AND BEYOND

The supplements in the Renew phase continue to strengthen and build upon the antioxidant protection, healthy cholesterol function, improved immune function, and the prebiotic and probiotic support for digestive health. This includes comprehensive multivitamin-multimineral support with ongoing prebiotic-probiotic protection that is essential to preserving the new healthy lifestyle you have built.

CVO (Cardiovascular Oil): A blend of high-quality krill oil with superior TG (triglyceride) fish oil, phytosterols, and coenzyme Q10 to support healthy cholesterol processes. The cholesterol sulfate in CVO is involved in cell membrane integrity and cardiovascular health. CVO is an excellent source of EPA and DHA omega-3 fatty acids, an important support for the ongoing health of your heart and gums.

Take 2 gel capsules twice a day with a meal.

Spectra One: *Continue to take 1 capsule twice a day.*

Spectra Two: *Take 1 dropper twice a day with Spectra One.*

FBR: *Take 1 or 2 scoops of powder in liquids or food once a day.*

MEDITATION (20 MINUTES AND BEYOND)

The goal is to lengthen your meditation time to twenty minutes. Once you are there, you might want to add another session. Two twenty-minute sessions of mindful meditation a day have been shown to reduce blood pressure and produce a relaxation response. Most of my patients find their meditation time a welcomed retreat from the endless demands of their lives. They say it makes them more effective in every way.

HIGH-INTENSITY WORKOUT (15 MINUTES TWICE A WEEK)

Continue with two fifteen-minute band workouts a week. If you find yourself going more than fifteen minutes to achieve muscle exhaustion, tighten up on the band to increase resistance. With more resistance, muscle failure will happen faster. It's like doing weight training with heavier weights.

RECREATION/MOVEMENT (BUILD TO 30 MINUTES MOST DAYS OF THE WEEK)

You should be a pro at building movement into your life by now. If you do not move enough, you will probably notice that you feel sluggish. That said, you can be a couch potato now and then. A day of rest is good for you.

RELAXATION POSTURES (10 MINUTES A DAY)

You may want to build to the full-body series so that you are releasing tension in all of your muscles, and you may find it helpful to do a specific posture at work now and then if you find tension mounting.

A Day on Week 4: Renew/ The New Lifestyle

Meditation (build to 20 minutes, and add another session if desired)*

Breakfast

Supplements with breakfast:

2 capsules CVO

2 scoops FBR

Snack

Supplements without food:

1 capsule Spectra One

1 dropper Spectra Two

Lunch

Recreation/Activity (30 minutes most days of the week)

Dinner

Supplement with dinner:

2 capsules CVO

Relaxation postures at least 40 minutes after dinner or before bed (10 minutes)†

Supplements without food:

1 capsule Spectra One

1 dropper Spectra Two

*Depending on what you prefer, you can meditate before dinner rather than in the morning.
†Relaxation techniques can be done before dinner or following workouts as well.

You are now adding grains, fruit, and sweet potatoes to your diet, which will give you a lot more range. Your options for smoothies expand, so check out the recipes. This week is an example of how to eat for the rest of your life.

The make-ahead recipes for Week 4 are:

Hearty Lentil Soup with Kale (see recipe page 247)
Red Quinoa Salad with a Crunch Factor (recipe page 275)
Yummy Oat Bars (recipe page 281)

Make sure you have enough Grace's Blast-Off Bars (recipe page 280), Peak Energy Trail Mix (recipe page 282), and Frittata Cupcakes (recipe pages 241–244) to get you through the week.

Day 1

Breakfast
Yogurt with fresh mixed berries

Midmorning snack
Peak Energy Trail Mix (recipe page 282)

Lunch
Vegetable Medley Quinoa (see recipe page 274)

Snack
Goji Almond Butter Truffles (recipe page 283)

Dinner
Guilt-Free Pizza of your choice (see recipe pages 262–264) with a
tossed salad

Day 2

Breakfast
Tropical Smoothie (recipe page 233)

Midmorning snack
Fresh figs in cream or with prosciutto

Lunch
Waldorf salad—chicken, apples, celery, walnuts, goji berries

Snack
Yummy Oat Bars (recipe page 281)

Dinner
Soy-Sesame Arctic Char (see recipe page 258)

Oven-Roasted Sweet Potato "Fries" (use recipe for Crispy Roasted Vegetables (recipe page 279))
Green Bean Salad with Red Quinoa (see recipe page 276)

Day 3

Breakfast
Basic Chia Cereal with diced apple (recipe page 240)

Midmorning snack
Bone Broth (recipe page 246)

Lunch
Vegetable Medley Quinoa leftovers (recipe page 274)

Snack
Cantaloupe wrapped in prosciutto or ham

Dinner
Hearty Lentil Soup with Kale (recipe page 247)

Day 4

Breakfast
2 Frittata Cupcakes (recipe pages 241–244)

Midmorning Snack
Apple slices with nut butter

Lunch
Tuna salad with celery, onions, and bell pepper in lettuce roll-up

Snack
Hummus with crudités

Dinner
French Green Lentils, Pears, and Shallot Salad with Arctic Char (see recipe page 265)

Day 5

Breakfast
Spinach and mushroom omelet with bacon

Snack
Pear slices with goat cheese

Lunch
Leftover Hearty Lentil Soup with Kale (page 247) over
Cauliflower Rice (page 272)

Snack
Yummy Oat Bars (page 281)

Dinner
Lemon Chicken with Sliced Almonds (see page 251)
Crispy Roasted Vegetables (page 279)

Day 6

Breakfast
Melon chunks with yogurt

Midmorning Snack
Bone Broth (page 246)

Lunch
Beef, turkey, chicken, or veggie burger with cheese of choice and
sautéed onions and mushrooms
Pickled vegetables

Snack
Strawberries in cream

Dinner
Seared or broiled sea scallops
Red Quinoa Salad with a Crunch Factor (see page 275)

Day 7

Breakfast
Poached or soft-boiled eggs on a bed of sautéed spinach with salsa

Midmorning Snack
An orange or clementine with nuts

Lunch
Leftover Red Quinoa Salad with a Crunch Factor (page 275)

Snack
  Yummy Oat Bars (recipe page 281)

Dinner
  Grilled or broiled steak
  Baked sweet potato with a maple syrup drizzle
  Green beans with sesame seeds and sesame oil

There you have it—a four-week plan that will help you reduce and eliminate killer inflammation and restore balance to your microbiome.

If you stick with my plan for a month, you will be elated by the results as my patients have been. By now, you are enjoying the subtle flavor of fresh, whole food. My patients tell me that the chemical tastes of colas, chips, and processed foods no longer appeal to them. Some say that the tastes of excessively sweet, salty, and fatty food have become disgusting to them. But no one is perfect 100 percent of the time. How could you pass up a piece of birthday cake at a surprise party given for you or a taste of family recipes for turkey dressing, lasagna, or holiday cookies? And don't forget pizza and a beer or a glass of wine after a long week.

Thanksgiving dinner is only a meal. Go for it! Controlled splurges are not going to hurt you. Indulge now and then and get right back on track. **If you can follow the program 80 percent of the time, you will be fine.**

If you are eating out at a fine restaurant, you don't have to pass up the dessert cart. Allow yourself to enjoy a rich dessert every now and then. Savor each forkful. You might find that a bite or two are all you need to feel satisfied. You don't have to inhale the whole treat. You can try eating half of what is served to you at any course and taking what remains on your plate home. You have to make a decision to go off the plan. If you are mindful about what you are eating, you will not lose control.

Some of my patients allow themselves to fall off the wagon, which is fine as long as they get back on again. They may go all out on a meal or two a week. One splurge meal or dessert is not going to destroy your health. Neither is a bad day. But it can be a slippery slope. An entire holiday season could become a problem. Your goal is to make a habit of eating well. When you stray, make the corrections you need quickly and get back on track.

As for exercise, recreation, and movement, I know you can get crazy busy. No matter what's going on, you can find a few minutes to meditate. If life is so hectic, you need ten minutes of relaxation postures. The fifteen-minute high-intensity band workout will make you feel more resilient. I have designed this program so that your time commitment is kept to a minimum. My advice is to do what you can, even if you have to reduce the time you can devote to restorative activities. You will feel better if you don't allow yourself to become sedentary or get tied up in knots of anxiety and stress. If you stray from the path, calm down and renew yourself.

Chapter Fourteen

When Needed

Refresh/Getting Back On Track

Your body changes all the time as it adjusts to the external and internal environment. A tight deadline, an ailing parent, a new job, too much partying during the holidays—there are so many situations that can distract you. Stressful times can throw off your equilibrium both emotionally and physically. This is when old cravings can resurface and your discipline can falter. Cravings for junk food will surface as you turn to "comfort" foods to make you feel better. Rather than lose the benefits you have gained, you have to take action. If you go off the plan for a stretch and find yourself consistently breaking the 80/20 rule by indulging too often in foods you know you should not be eating, go back to Week 1.

You have to refresh your resolve to take care of yourself. You don't have to start over. You just have to refresh your efforts. Your goal at this point is to reestablish the bidirectional connections: gut/oral, gut/brain/oral, gut/immune.

SUPPLEMENTS FOR THE REFRESH PHASE

The supplements reintroduced in the Refresh phase are designed to reengage neurological control, repair glucose metabolic functions, and probiotic proliferation. These should be taken for one to two weeks along with your regular supplementation with Spectra One, Spectra Two, CVO, and FBR. This is the drill:

Synulin: To repair glucose metabolism and reduce the renewed sugar/carb cravings.

Take 1 capsule twice daily.

Neurosyn: To reengage neurological control.

Take 1 capsule twice daily.

MBC: To reestablish a healthy probiotic proliferation.

Take 2 to 4 capsules daily with food.

Chapter Fifteen

Superfood Recipes for Balance

When I started to think about what recipes to include in *The Mouth⇔Body Connection*, I found myself thinking about the superfoods. Though the foods on my list are high in nutritional value, many of them are on the cutting edge of food trends. I decided it would be a good idea to give you an idea of the range of these foods. I do not want you to feel that the Triple A Diet is about deprivation.

You can do amazing things with your protein shakes that will make them seem sinful, though they are not. Experimenting with lacto-fermented vegetables will open a whole new world of food preparation for you as you prepare your own probiotic food. Eggs are a great source of protein. I want to give you a few recipes to prepare ahead, such as Frittata Cupcakes, which you can have on hand in the freezer. Chia seeds make sweet and savory cereals and puddings that you will enjoy if you haven't already. I have included a basic bone broth recipe, because of the soup's remineralizing effect. You might want to get in the habit of sipping on bone broth throughout the day. And of course, there is Healing Chicken Soup. If you have been chickened to death in recent years, you will enjoy the recipes I've included for chicken breasts, because they use many of the other superfoods on the list. You may not be familiar with Arctic char or are reluctant to prepare fish. The delicious recipes included in this chapter will make you a convert. Would you like to eat pizza without guilt? You'll find the answer in the coming pages. And did you ever think mashed potatoes or rice would be on your plate again? That wonderful vegetable cauliflower will make it all possible. Interesting salads and tasty treats finish the selections. From a Red Velvet Shake to Let the Good Times Roll Spicy Pecan Chicken, from Tropical Kale Chips to Goji Almond Butter Truffles, you will find delectable recipes that are easy to make and that will open your eyes to the abundance of healthy choices out there for you. Once you start eating this way, you will feel and look so good, you will want to leave your old habits far behind.

SUPERFOODS RECIPE LIST

SMOOTHIES (page 230)

Dr. Gerry's Super Smile Smoothie
Double Chocolate Protein Shake
What to Do with Leftover Coffee Shake
Red Velvet Shake
Mocha Boost
Berry, Berry Antioxidant Shake
Free Radical Eradicator
Tropical Smoothie

LACTO-FERMENTED VEGETABLES (page 234)

Salsa with a Kick
Old-Fashioned Dill Pickled Green Beans
Tangy Grape Tomatoes
Spring in a Jar: Asparagus Pickle
Spicy Brussels Sprouts
Snappy Pickled Celery Sticks

BREAKFAST (page 240)

Basic Chia Cereal
Chia Goji Berry Breakfast Pudding
Sun-Dried Tomato, Basil, and Goat Cheese Frittata Cupcakes
Asparagus Artichoke Frittata Cupcakes
Vegetable Medley Frittata Cupcakes

SOUP (page 246)

Basic Bone Broth
Hearty Lentil Soup with Kale
Healing Chicken Soup
Chicken Zoodle Detox Soup

CHICKEN (page 250)

Chicken Marsala
Lemon Chicken with Sliced Almonds
Coconut Chicken Breasts
Stir-Fry Chicken with Broccoli
Curried Chicken Salad in Lettuce Packages
Broiled Country Mustard Chicken
Let the Good Times Roll Spicy Pecan Chicken

ARCTIC CHAR (page 257)

Georgia's Pistachio-Crusted Arctic Char with Steamed Broccoli
Soy-Sesame Arctic Char
Baked Arctic Char with a Scallion Crust
Garlic-Dill Baked Char
Cajun Blackened Arctic Char

MAIN COURSE (page 261)

Meatless or Meaty Chili
Variations on Guilt-Free Pizza

Roasted Vegetables and Goat Cheese
Gorgonzola and Caramelized Onion Pizza
Fontina and Mushroom Pizza with a Fried Egg
French Green Lentils, Pears, and Shallot Salad with Arctic Char

CAULIFLOWER (page 267)

Mediterranean Oven-Roasted Cauliflower
Brown Butter Drizzled Cauliflower Steaks
Lemon Parsley Roasted Cauliflower
I Can't Believe It's Not Mashed Potatoes
Variation on Mashed Cauliflower
Centerpiece Cauliflower
A Sauce Option
"Kill Your Carb Craving" Cauliflower Rice Basic Recipe
Cauliflower Fried Rice

SALADS (page 274)

Quinoa: The Perfect "Grain" as a Blank Canvas
Vegetable Medley Quinoa
Red Quinoa Salad with a Crunch Factor
Green Bean Salad with Red Quinoa
Cucumber and Celery Refresher
Superfood Special: Kale, Avocado, and Olive Salad

SNACKS (page 279)

Crispy Roasted Vegetables
Tropical Kale Chips
Grace's Blast-Off Bars
Yummy Oat Bars
Peak Energy Trail Mix
Goji Almond Butter Truffles
Coconut Bliss Balls

S M O O T H I E S

Protein shakes are a good option for busy people, especially for breakfast. You can use protein powder and water or unsweetened nut milk, shake it up, and that's it. You can also turn your smoothies into a treat and increase the anti-inflammatory nutrients you consume as you drink your shake. The possibilities are limitless. Here are just a few examples to get you going. The sky is the limit here—be creative!

Dr. Gerry's Super Smile Smoothie

Serves 1

This is the shake I have every morning. I sometimes forget it's time for lunch, because this smoothie is full of good fats and protein and I do not get hungry. Starting the day with this nutritious launch keeps my energy level even and propels me through my busy schedule.

> 1 scoop RH Dynamic Fruits & Greens*
> 1 scoop collagen protein powder (non-GMO)
> ½ cup ice cubes
> 1 cup mixed frozen berries (can be added on Week 4)
> 1 cup organic unsweetened coconut milk (to cover ingredients)

Put the dry ingredients, ice, and berries in a blender. Cover with the coconut milk. Blend until smooth.

*This powder delivers the antioxidant power of twenty fruits and vegetables. There are many Super Green powders available, but this is the one I use and recommend.

Double Chocolate Protein Shake

Serves 1

If you are a chocoholic, this is the shake for you. Simple and densely chocolate, this shake will help to satisfy your sweet cravings.

1 scoop chocolate protein powder

1 cup water, whole milk, or unsweetened almond milk

2½ tablespoons unsweetened cacao powder

2 ice cubes

Combine all the ingredients in a blender, and blend until smooth.

What to Do with Leftover Coffee Shake

Serves 1

Don't pour the coffee left in your pot down the drain. Use it in a delicious shake that you can enjoy any time of day. This shake is a pick-me-up that also delivers a dose of protein.

1 scoop vanilla protein powder

1 cup cold coffee

3 ice cubes

Combine all the ingredients in a blender, and blend until smooth.

Red Velvet Shake

Serves 1

Do you miss sweet desserts? If you do, this Red Velvet Shake will fit the bill. Beets are sweet vegetables, so don't overdo it.

1 scoop chocolate protein powder

1 cup water or unsweetened almond milk

1 small beet, peeled and boiled until tender

Combine all the ingredients in a blender, and blend until smooth.

Mocha Boost

Serves 1

This is a supercharged smoothie that tastes as if a *barista* created it just for you.

1 scoop chocolate protein powder
½ cup cold water or unsweetened almond milk
1 teaspoon granulated instant coffee
5 ice cubes

Combine the first three ingredients in a blender.
   Add the ice cubes gradually, and blend to the desired consistency.

Berry, Berry Antioxidant Shake

(Week 4)

Serves 1

Creamy as can be, this shake has staying power. Using yogurt or coconut cream in your shake will produce a creamier smoothie. It will fill you up and please your palate at the same time. Experiment with different combinations of fruit. You should hold off on this shake until Week 4.

1 scoop vanilla protein powder
1 cup blackberries
½ cup water
½ cup plain Greek yogurt
½ cup blueberries
water and/or ice

Combine the first five ingredients in a blender.
   Add ice or water gradually, and blend to the desired consistency.

Free Radical Eradicator

(Week 4)

Serves 1

This antioxidant smoothie is a delicious anti-aging elixir. The cashews and the avocado provide healthy fats, and the dried goji berries plus fresh or frozen berries neutralize oxidative stress. Do not be tempted to enjoy this smoothie before Week 4 of the program, when you can incorporate fruit into your daily diet.

1½ cups filtered water or unsweetened almond milk

2 tablespoons raw cashews

2 tablespoons goji berries

1 cup fresh or frozen strawberries, raspberries, or blueberries or a combination

½ avocado

In a blender, pulse the water or almond milk and cashews until creamy.
    Add the goji berries, frozen or fresh berries, and avocado, and blend until smooth.

Tropical Smoothie

(Week 4)

Serves 1

Close your eyes when you take a sip of this smoothie and you will think you are on a beach or sitting poolside at a four-star resort in Hawaii, Mexico, or the Caribbean. The Vitamin C content of this smoothie is through the roof.

¼ cup fresh or frozen strawberries

¼ cup fresh or frozen pineapple, papaya, or mango

¼ cup dried goji berries

juice of 1 lime

1½ cups coconut water to cover ingredients

Combine all the ingredients in a blender, and blend until smooth.

LACTO-FERMENTED VEGETABLES

When you ferment your vegetables, you are creating healthy probiotics to help balance your microbiome. Since fermentation takes time, you have to plan for it. You have to prepare these vegetables in advance, but they are worth the wait. I will list the fermentation time for each recipe so that you can plan ahead.

You should stock up on some mason jars and start to save the jars you would normally discard. Running the repurposed jars through the dishwasher is enough to clean them for their new use.

I like to use freeze-dried starter cultures, because they can speed the process. You can find them online and in the health food department of most good supermarkets and health food stores. Except for one recipe, these vegetables require a brine made of salt and water.

Salt Brine for Lacto Fermentation

6 tablespoons fine sea salt or 9 tablespoons coarse sea salt
8 cups filtered water

Mix together.

Salsa with a Kick

Serves 6–8

Fermenting time: 3–4 days

You can whip this condiment together in no time, and nothing is easier to incorporate into your diet than salsa. On eggs, chicken, fish, burgers, or as a dip—salsa will liven up anything you are eating. Taking the time to ferment store-bought salsa will increase the nutritional value exponentially.

You will be creating healthy probiotics that will keep your microbiome in balance. The good news is that you can keep lacto-fermented vegetables in a covered jar for weeks in the refrigerator.

16-ounce container fresh organic salsa or *pico de gallo* from the refrigerated section of the supermarket
2 tablespoons starter culture

Pour the salsa or *pico de gallo* into a pint-size mason jar.
Stir in the starter culture.
Cover with a loosely closed lid, dishcloth, paper towel, or coffee filter, and secure with a rubber band.
Let the salsa ferment at room temperature for 2 to 3 days, then seal and refrigerate.
When sealed with a cap and refrigerated, this salsa will keep for weeks or months.

Old-Fashioned Dill Pickled Green Beans

Yield: 1 quart
Serves 6–8

Fermenting time: 1–2 weeks

Pickled beans are a throwback to a time when produce was not available year round. Think *Little House on the Prairie*. The fact is that pickled beans are delicious and are great in a salad, as a snack, or as a side dish at lunch or dinner.

4 cups organic green beans
3 cloves garlic, peeled and halved
1 tablespoon dill seed or 3 tablespoons fresh dill
2–3 cups sea salt and water brine (page 234)

Snap the ends off the green beans and wash them.
Place the garlic and dill in 1 quart jar or 2 pint jars.
Stand the green beans upright in the jar, leaving at least 1 inch of headspace. Be sure to pack the beans in tightly.
Pour in brine to 1 inch from the top of the jar.
Loosely lid or cover the jar and let it sit at room temperature for at least 3 days. Check to see if the beans have reached the desired level of sourness.

When the beans are ready, close the jar with a tight lid and refrigerate. If they need more time fermenting, leave the jar out until the beans pass the taste test. The beans are usually tastiest after they have fermented between 1 and 2 weeks.

Tangy Grape Tomatoes

Yield: 1 quart
Serves 10–12

Fermenting time: 3 days to 2 weeks, depending on level of sourness desired

Tomatoes and basil are a great flavor combination. These fermented tomatoes make for a tasty snack, side dish, or salad ingredient. They can be great with small balls of mozzarella. We always have a jar in our refrigerator.

1 quart grape tomatoes
1 bunch fresh basil
4 cups filtered water
3 tablespoons Celtic Sea Salt

Wash the tomatoes.

Make a hole in each tomato with a toothpick, which will allow the brine to penetrate the tomatoes.

Put a layer of tomatoes at the bottom of a 1-quart, wide-mouthed canning jar.

Place one or two basil leaves on top of the tomatoes.

Keep layering the tomatoes and the basil until the jar is filled up within 1½ inches from the mouth.

Mix the water with the Celtic Sea Salt.

Pour the brine over the tomatoes, leaving 1 inch of space at the top.

Use a glass canning lid, a small bag filled with brine, or a well-scrubbed stone to keep the tomatoes from floating.

Cover the jar loosely with a dish towel to allow the gas to escape.

Place the jar in a dark place such as a cupboard or a kitchen cabinet for at least 3 to 5 days. Taste for the degree of sourness you enjoy.

When the tomatoes pass the taste test, cover the jar with a lid and refrigerate.

Spring in a Jar: Asparagus Pickle

Yield: 1 quart

Serves 6–8

Fermenting time: 5–8 days

1–2 pounds asparagus spears

3–4 cloves garlic

1 tablespoon black peppercorns

½ teaspoon chili pepper flakes

1 bay leaf

3–4 dried red chiles (cayenne for spicy; sweet for color in the jar
without heat)

2–3 cups brine

To make the brine, mix together:

¾ cup unrefined sea salt

1 gallon filtered water

You can store any leftover brine in the refrigerator. It will keep for a
week. Discard after 7 days.

Snap the woody ends off the asparagus spears. Cut the spears so
that they can stand upright in a 1-quart jar. A length of about 5 inches
leaves room for the brine to cover them.

Crush the garlic cloves with the flat side of a knife.

Place the peppercorns, pepper flakes, and a bay leaf in the bottom of
the jar.

Arrange the spears upright and wedge the garlic and dried chiles
between them.

Pour in brine to 1 inch from the top of the jar.

Cover loosely with the jar lid, dish towel, or paper towel closed with a
rubber band.

Put the jar on a baking sheet to ferment, in a cool place out of direct
light for 5 to 8 days. Keep an eye on the brine level and make sure the
asparagus are completely covered. If they are not, top off with the
reserved brine solution.

You may see scum on top; it's generally harmless, but you will want
to skim it off.

When the brine is cloudy and the spears are a dull olive green, the
pickles are ready.

Tighten the lid and store the jar in the refrigerator. After a day, check to see if the pickles are still submerged. Top off with reserved brine, if needed.

The refrigerated asparagus pickles will keep for 12 months. The flavor will intensify over time.

Spicy Brussels Sprouts

Serves 6–8

Fermenting time: 1–2 weeks

Since Brussels sprouts have such rich flavor, they are perfect for fermenting.

  4–5 garlic cloves

  1 tablespoon whole peppercorns

  1 tablespoon chili pepper flakes

  1 pound Brussels sprouts, halved

  2–3 jalapeños, cut into strips or rounds, or 2 tablespoons canned or jarred rounds

  salt brine (page 234)

For extra flavor, you might want to try a smoky brine:

  ½ gallon filtered water

  2 tablespoons unrefined sea salt

  2 tablespoons smoked salt

Place the garlic cloves, peppercorns, and chili pepper flakes in the bottom of a 1-quart jar.

Arrange the Brussels sprouts and the jalapeños in layers to just below the shoulder of the jar.

Cover the Brussels sprouts with brine. Keep leftover brine in the refrigerator, for up to a week.

Put a piece of plastic wrap over the Brussels sprouts. Put a sealed, water-filled Ziploc bag on top of the plastic to keep the vegetables in place.

Put the jar on a baking sheet in a cool place without direct sunlight for 7 to 14 days.

Check the level of the brine regularly. If the vegetables are not covered, add more brine solution until the liquid completely covers the Brussels sprouts.

As the vegetables ferment, their color fades and the brine gets cloudy. At this point, just when you hit a week, you can start to test your pickles. When the sprouts are sour enough for your taste, they are done.

Tighten the lid and refrigerate. The Brussels sprouts will keep for 6 months in the refrigerator.

Snappy Pickled Celery Sticks

Yield: 12–20 pickles

Cooling time: 2 hours

What is great about this recipe is that the celery doesn't have to sit in the pickling juice for days. Your pickled celery will be ready to serve in just 2 hours. They are great in salads and wraps and make a fine garnish.

8 large celery stalks, peeled
1 cup white vinegar
1 teaspoon powdered or liquid organic stevia
salt to taste
4 garlic cloves, smashed
1 tablespoon mustard seeds
1 teaspoon red chili flakes
1 tablespoon cracked peppercorns

Cut the celery to the height of your mason jar.

Bring the vinegar, stevia, and salt to a boil in a small saucepan. Stir until the powdered stevia and salt are dissolved. Remove from the heat and add the garlic, mustard seeds, chili flakes, and peppercorns.

Put the pieces of celery upright in a tall, wide-mouthed mason jar and pour the liquid over the celery. Cover the jar tightly.

If you prefer, you can put the celery in a large ceramic or glass bowl and pour the vinegar mixture over the celery.

As the pickles cool, gently shake the jar to distribute the spices and brine.

Allow the pickles to cool completely before serving.

BREAKFAST

Starting your day with a wholesome breakfast rather than a pastry will boost your energy and lower your appetite for the entire day. Since eggs are a superfood and you are welcome to have bacon on the Triple A Diet, you can have a hearty breakfast each day. In addition, the recipes that follow can be prepared ahead of time. They will allow you to eat well without having to deal with making breakfast in the morning.

Basic Chia Cereal

Serves 2

For a tiny seed, chia packs a nutritional wallop. Chia is low-carb. In fact, most of the carbs found in the seeds are fiber. They are high in antioxidants and minerals, including calcium, magnesium, and phosphorus, which are key to the health of your teeth and your bones. They are an excellent source of protein and omega-3s as well. When wet chia seeds become gelatinous and create a "pudding," I consider chia cereal to be a healthier alternative to oatmeal, and it's quicker to make. You can dress it up just as you would oatmeal—with cinnamon, nutmeg, nuts, and fruit in any combination.

- 1 cup chia seeds
- 1 teaspoon butter from grass-bred cows
- 1 tablespoon coconut oil
- 1 teaspoon goji berries
- 1 teaspoon chopped dates or prunes (optional)
- 1 teaspoon shredded coconut, pumpkin seeds, or chopped nuts (optional)
- ½ cup filtered water

Put all the ingredients in a small bowl and add the water.

Allow the mixture to sit for 5 minutes. When it is gelatinous, stir the contents of the bowl and serve. If the mixture is too thick, add more water.

You can refrigerate leftovers for a day or two.

Chia Goji Berry Breakfast Pudding

Serves 1

Gelling time: 30 minutes or overnight

A breakfast pudding might seem exotic to you, but I think you could get used to it very quickly because it tastes so good. This recipe produces a richer, creamier pudding. One of the pluses is that you can make it the night before you plan to eat it, so you do not have to fuss with preparing breakfast.

Chia Pudding

> ½ cup unsweetened almond milk
> 2 tablespoons white or black chia seeds
> ½ teaspoon vanilla extract
> ½ teaspoon ground cinnamon

Toppings

> 2 tablespoons goldenberries
> 2 tablespoons goji berries
> 2 tablespoons dried mulberries
> 2 tablespoons raw cashews
> 1 teaspoon raw cacao nibs (optional)
> 2 tablespoons fresh berries (after Week 4)

Pour the almond milk over the chia seeds. Whisk well with a fork, making sure to break up any clumps.

Whisk in the vanilla extract and cinnamon.

Let sit for 5 minutes, stir again, and place in the refrigerator for 30 minutes or overnight.

After 30 minutes or the next morning, top with berries and cashews.

Sun-Dried Tomato, Basil, and Goat Cheese Frittata Cupcakes

Yield: 10–12 cupcakes
Serves: 5–12

Frittata Cupcakes make a terrific breakfast, lunch, or snack. What is great about them is that you can make a batch, wrap each individually, and freeze them in a bag or covered bowl. Without much effort, you can have a week's worth of breakfasts and/or snacks. I like to have an emergency supply in the freezer for when I am in a rush.

5 or 6 sun-dried tomatoes

½ cup packed fresh basil leaves

6 cage-free eggs

3 tablespoons filtered water

¼ teaspoon sea salt

¼ teaspoon pepper

2 scallions, thinly sliced white parts and most of the green

2 tablespoons extra virgin olive oil

4 ounces fresh white goat cheese, crumbled

Preheat the oven to 350 degrees.

In a medium bowl, cover the tomatoes in very hot tap water and soak them for 5–15 minutes to soften and plump them.

Drain and thinly slice the tomatoes.

Make a basil chiffonade by stacking the basil leaves in batches, rolling the stacks cigarette-style, and slicing across into thin ribbons.

In a large bowl, whisk the eggs, filtered water, salt, and pepper until frothy.

Stir in the scallions.

Spray olive oil into a nonstick cupcake tin, or you can also use cupcake papers in the tin.

Add the egg mixture, sun-dried tomatoes, goat cheese, and basil.

Bake 15–20 minutes or until eggs are completely set.

Allow the frittatas to cool. Gently remove from the pan using a spoon.

Garnish with any remaining basil and goat cheese.

After cooling, you can wrap each frittata individually and freeze them in a plastic bag or covered bowl. Just warm them up in the oven or a microwave and you are good to go.

Asparagus Artichoke Frittata Cupcakes

Serves 4–6

Here is another knockout combination for your frittata cupcake.

2½ tablespoons extra virgin olive oil

½ yellow onion, diced

6 eggs

3 tablespoons water

¼ teaspoon sea salt

¼ teaspoon pepper

6 artichoke hearts, cut into quarters

1 bunch asparagus, with woody stems removed, cut into 1-inch pieces

½ cup packed fresh basil leaves

Preheat the oven to 350 degrees.

In a nonstick frying pan, add ½ tablespoon olive oil and cook the onion over medium heat until translucent.

In a large bowl, whisk the eggs, water, salt, and pepper until frothy. Stir in the onion.

In a 10-inch nonstick skillet, heat 2 tablespoons olive oil over high heat. Add the artichoke hearts and pieces of asparagus. Cook for 2 minutes. Reduce the heat to medium. Add the basil and cook for 2 minutes longer, until heated but still bright in color.

Spoon this mixture into a nonstick cupcake pan and pour the egg mixture over the vegetables.

Bake 15–20 minutes or until eggs are set.

Another option:

If you want to make a meal-sized frittata:

Instead of using a cupcake tin, keep the vegetables in the skillet and pour the eggs over them. Cook for 1 minute, until the edges set slightly.

Cover, reduce heat to very low, and cook about 20 minutes or until the center of the frittata is set but still moist.

Turn out the frittata onto a dinner plate, then invert to a second plate, top side up.

Serve hot or at room temperature, cut into wedges.

Vegetable Medley Frittata Cupcakes

Yield: 12 cupcakes

Once you get used to making these frittatas, you can use the eggs as a medium for incorporating more vegetables into your diet. You can come up with any combination of vegetables that you like and use any shredded cheese you want. I think this combo is very, very good.

   5 tablespoons extra virgin olive oil

   1 onion, chopped

   3 garlic cloves, minced

   ¼ cup dry white wine

   1 red bell pepper, chopped

   2 celery ribs, chopped

   ½ pound fresh mushrooms, sliced

   1 medium tomato, seeded and chopped

   1 tablespoon chopped fresh thyme, basil, oregano, parsley, and/or chives

   ½ teaspoon sea salt

   ¼ teaspoon pepper

   6 eggs

   3 tablespoons whole milk or unsweetened almond milk

   1 cup shredded mozzarella or provolone cheese

Preheat the oven to 350 degrees.

In a medium frying pan, heat 3 tablespoons of extra virgin olive oil over medium-high heat. Add the onion and cook, stirring occasionally, until softened, about 3 minutes.

Add the garlic and stir for two minutes.

Pour in the wine and boil over high heat until evaporated to about 1 tablespoon, about 2 minutes. Transfer to a large mixing bowl, and wipe out the frying pan.

In the same pan, heat the remaining 2 tablespoons of olive oil over medium-high heat.

Add the bell pepper and celery and cook, stirring until softened, about 3 minutes.

Add the mushrooms and cook 3 minutes longer.

Add the tomato and herbs. Cook until the mixture is dry, about 4 minutes.

Season with ¼ teaspoon salt and ⅛ teaspoon pepper.

Add the vegetables to the onion and mix well.

Put the vegetables in the bottom of each cupcake paper in a cupcake pan or straight into a nonstick cupcake pan you have rubbed with olive oil.

In a medium bowl, whisk the eggs, milk, and the remaining salt and pepper until blended. Pour the egg mix evenly over the vegetables.

Bake for 15 minutes. Remove from the oven and sprinkle the cheese over the top of each cupcake.

Return to the oven and bake for 10–15 minutes, until the cupcakes are almost set but jiggly in the center.

Let cool on a wire rack for 5 minutes.

Wrap and freeze any leftover cupcakes.

S O U P

I have focused on both broth and chicken soup in this section, and have thrown in a lentil and kale soup for good measure. I want to drive home the point that you should make bone broth a regular part of your diet. You need those oral health building minerals.

Basic Bone Broth

Yield: 1–2 gallons

Simmer time:

Beef—48 hours

Poultry—24 hours

Fish—8 hours

If you are concerned about leaving the broth simmering on a stovetop, use a slow cooker on low or medium.

It's a good idea to always have bone broth in your freezer. You can freeze the broth in ice cube trays and transfer them to a plastic bag once frozen. Storing broth this way makes it easy to use it in your everyday cooking, whenever stock is called for in a recipe. Bone broth is very nutritious. Rather than taking a coffee break, bring a thermos of bone broth to the office or warm up a bowl at home to sip throughout the day. The broth is nutritious (page 111) and satisfying.

- 2–4 pounds bones from a healthy source—use bones from only one source for each broth: beef, poultry, or fish
- 1–2 gallons filtered water—aim for 2 pounds of bones per gallon of water
- 3 tablespoons apple cider vinegar
- 1 onion, quartered
- 3 large carrots, roughly chopped
- 2 stalks of celery, roughly chopped
- 1 tablespoon Celtic Sea Salt
- Optional: 1 teaspoon peppercorns, additional herbs or spices; 1 bunch parsley, fresh herbs, and 2 cloves garlic added for the last 30 minutes

Preheat the oven to 350 degrees if you are using raw bones.

Roast the bones for 30 minutes in a roasting pan, which will improve the flavor.

Place the bones in a large stockpot and pour the water and the vinegar over the bones. Let the bones sit for 20–30 minutes in the cool water, which makes the nutrients in the bones more available.

Add the vegetables to the pot along with the salt, pepper, herbs, and spices.

Bring the broth to a boil, then reduce the heat to a simmer and cook for:

Beef broth: 48 hours

Poultry broth: 24 hours

Fish broth: 8 hours

Make certain the burner is on low heat and that nothing flammable is near the stockpot. You can also use a slow cooker to make bone broth.

During the first 2 hours of simmering, a frothy foam will float on the surface of the broth. This can be scooped out with a big spoon and discarded.

Add the fresh parsley, herbs, and garlic for the last 30 minutes.

When finished, remove from heat and let cool slightly. Strain, using a fine metal strainer, to remove the bones and the vegetables.

When cool, store in a covered glass jar or bowl in the refrigerator for up to 5 days, or freeze for later use.

Hearty Lentil Soup with Kale

Serves 6

When you are cooking this stick-to-your-ribs soup, your kitchen will smell wonderful. With a salad or pickled vegetables on the side, it's a nutrition-packed main course. It freezes well—so make a big batch.

    1 tablespoon extra virgin olive oil

    4 leeks, white and light green parts, cut into ¼-inch-thick slices

    1 (28-ounce) can whole organic tomatoes, drained

    6 cups filtered water

    2 sweet potatoes, peeled and cut into ½-inch pieces

    1 bunch kale, thick stems removed and leaves cut into ½-inch-wide strips

    ½ cup brown lentils

    1 tablespoon fresh thyme

    kosher salt and black pepper

    ¼ cup or 1 ounce grated Parmesan cheese

Heat the oil in a large saucepan or Dutch oven over medium heat.

Add the leeks and cook, stirring occasionally, until they begin to soften, 3 to 4 minutes.

Add the tomatoes and cook, breaking them up with a spoon, 5 minutes. Add 6 cups of filtered water and bring to a boil.

Stir in the sweet potatoes, kale, lentils, thyme, 1½ teaspoons salt, and ¼ teaspoon pepper.

Simmer until the lentils are tender, 25–30 minutes.

Spoon into bowls and top with the Parmesan cheese.

Healing Chicken Soup

Serves 6–8

If chicken soup makes you feel better when you are sick, imagine what it will do for you when you are well. Chicken soup is the ultimate comfort food. Don't wait until you are sick to have some.

This recipe is as basic as it can be. If you'd like, you can add a cup of cooked quinoa, some steamed vegetables, or a handful of spinach or kale to the soup.

When you are in Week 1, Healing Chicken Soup will support your detox. Nothing is more comforting than steaming homemade chicken soup.

3½- to 4-pound chicken

6 carrots, peeled

4 celery stalks, trimmed

1 large yellow onion, quartered

1½ teaspoons Celtic Sea Salt

1 teaspoon whole black peppercorns

8 cups filtered water

Place the chicken in a large pot.

Cut 4 carrots and 2 celery stalks into 1-inch pieces. Add with the onion to the pot.

Add the salt, peppercorns, and enough cold filtered water to cover the chicken, about 8 cups.

Bring to a boil. Reduce the heat and simmer, skimming any foam that rises to the top, until the chicken is cooked through, about 30 minutes.

Transfer the chicken to a bowl and let cool.

Strain the broth and discard the vegetables.

Return the broth to the pot.

Thinly slice the remaining carrots and celery and add to the broth. Simmer until tender, about 10 minutes.

When the chicken is cool enough to handle, shred the meat and add it to the soup.

Chicken Zoodle Detox Soup

Serves 6

If you miss those noodles, this recipe is the answer. This recipe requires a spiralizer, which will allow you to make noodles from vegetables. When spiralizing zucchini, you create "zoodles."

2 tablespoons extra virgin olive oil

1 pound boneless, organic skinless chicken breasts, cut into 1-inch chunks

kosher salt and freshly ground black pepper

3 cloves garlic, minced

1 onion, diced

3 carrots, peeled and diced

2 stalks celery, diced

½ teaspoon dried thyme

¼ teaspoon dried rosemary

4 cups salt-free organic chicken stock

1 bay leaf

2 cups filtered water

1 pound or 3 medium-size zucchini, spiralized

2 tablespoons freshly squeezed lemon juice

1 sprig rosemary

2 tablespoons chopped fresh parsley leaves

Heat 1 tablespoon olive oil in a large stockpot or Dutch oven over medium heat.

Season the chicken with salt and pepper to taste.

Add the chicken to the stockpot, toss for 2 minutes until golden. Remove the chicken and set it aside.

Add the remaining 1 tablespoon olive oil to the stockpot. Add the garlic, onion, carrots, and celery. Cook, stirring occasionally, until tender, about 3–4 minutes.

Stir in the thyme and rosemary until fragrant, about 1 minute.

Whisk in the chicken stock, bay leaf, and water and bring to a boil.

Stir in the zucchini noodles and chicken. Reduce the heat and simmer until the zucchini is tender, about 3–5 minutes.

Stir in the lemon juice. Season with salt and pepper to taste.

Serve immediately, garnished with fresh rosemary and parsley.

C H I C K E N

You will be eating a lot of chicken on this program. It's a good thing chicken is so versatile! Nothing could be easier than roasting a chicken, and you can get a few meals out of it. Or you could buy a rotisserie chicken, have it for dinner, and use the leftovers sliced for lunch, in chicken salad, or in chicken broth. I have focused on boneless chicken breasts here, because cooking time is reduced.

Chicken Marsala

Serves 4

Chicken Marsala is a wonderful Italian dish. One of the joys of the Triple A Diet is that you can have butter and a bit of heavy cream. This chicken is like velvet.

> 4 tablespoons butter or extra virgin olive oil or half of each
> 4 skinless, boneless chicken breast halves, pounded to ¼-inch thickness
> 4 shallots, finely chopped
> ½ pound mushrooms, sliced
> ¼ cup dry Marsala
> ½ cup heavy cream
> 1 teaspoon lemon juice
> sea salt and freshly ground pepper to taste

In a large frying pan, melt 2 tablespoons butter or warm olive oil over medium heat.

Add the chicken and sauté, turning once, until lightly browned, about 2 minutes on each side. Remove and set aside.

Melt the remaining butter or warm the olive oil in the same pan.

Add the shallots and mushrooms. Cook until the mushrooms are lightly browned, 3–5 minutes.

Add the Marsala and bring to a boil, scraping up any browned bits from the bottom of the pan.

Add the cream and lemon juice and return to a boil.

Season with salt and pepper to taste.

Return the chicken to the pan and cook, turning in the sauce, for about 3 minutes to reheat and finish cooking.

Lemon Chicken with Sliced Almonds

Serves 6

Marinating time: 1 hour

This is a modern take on the classic French recipe for Chicken Almandine. The dish works well with green beans and cauliflower rice. The finished product presents well, so it's a great company dish. Everyone (who does not have a nut allergy) loves it!

6 skinless, boneless chicken breast halves, pounded to ¼-inch thickness
⅓ cup lemon juice
3 tablespoons Dijon mustard
2 garlic cloves, finely chopped
¼ teaspoon freshly ground pepper
⅓ cup extra virgin olive oil
½ cup sliced almonds
2 tablespoons butter
1 cup no-salt organic chicken broth
1 teaspoon coconut or almond flour as a substitute for the traditional cornstarch
2 tablespoons chopped fresh parsley
¼ teaspoon cayenne pepper
lemon slices, for garnish

Place the chicken breasts in a large, shallow baking dish.

Combine the lemon juice, mustard, garlic, and pepper in a small bowl. Beat in the olive oil. Pour over the chicken. Marinate 1 hour at room temperature.

Preheat the oven to 350 degrees.

Place the almonds in a small baking pan. Bake until lightly browned, about 10 minutes.

Drain the chicken and reserve the marinade.

In a large frying pan, melt the butter over medium heat. Add the chicken and cook about 4 minutes on each side, until lightly browned. Remove the chicken to a dish.

Add the reserved marinade and the chicken broth to the pan. Boil over high heat, stirring, until the sauce reduces by half, about 5 minutes. Stir in the coconut or almond flour and cook, stirring, until thickened and smooth. Add the parsley and cayenne pepper.

Reduce the heat, return the chicken to the pan, and heat through.

Transfer the chicken to a serving platter and pour the sauce over it. Sprinkle toasted almonds over the chicken and garnish with lemon slices.

Coconut Chicken Breasts

Serves 6

A Caribbean treat, chicken breasts with coconut and a touch of brown sugar are a simple way to make a flavorful statement that will transform your go-to protein. I can almost hear the steel drums in the background when I eat this dish.

    6 skinless, boneless chicken breast halves
    sea salt and freshly ground pepper
    4 tablespoons butter
    2 tablespoons extra virgin coconut oil
    2 sweet onions, thinly sliced
    1 tablespoon brown sugar
    ¼ cup roasted red peppers, slivered
    3 tablespoons raisins
    3 teaspoons lemon juice
    ¾ cup flaked coconut
    3 teaspoons chopped parsley

Preheat the oven to 375 degrees.

Season chicken with salt and pepper.

In a large frying pan, melt 2 tablespoons butter and 2 tablespoons coconut oil over medium heat.

Add the chicken and cook until lightly browned, about 3 minutes a side. Transfer the chicken to an 8-by-12-by-2-inch baking dish.

Add the onions to the same frying pan and cook until soft, 3–5 minutes.

Add the brown sugar, red peppers, raisins, 1½ teaspoons lemon juice, and 1½ teaspoons of parsley. Pour the mixture over the chicken and cover with foil. Bake 10 minutes.

While the chicken is baking, melt the remaining 2 tablespoons butter.

In a small bowl, combine the melted butter, coconut, 1½ teaspoons lemon juice, 1½ teaspoons parsley, ½ teaspoon salt, and ¼ teaspoon pepper.

Return the chicken to the frying pan and cover with the sauce. Turn the chicken breasts in the sauce to coat. Simmer 5–10 minutes until the chicken is tender.

Remove the chicken to a serving platter and spoon the sauce over it.

Stir-Fry Chicken with Broccoli

Serves 4

Stir-frying is an easy way to toss a healthy meal together. I am including one recipe, but you can use any protein and whatever combination of vegetables you like. I like steak, shrimp, or scallops tossed in a wok or frying pan with vegetables. Water chestnuts and sprouts are good for crunch. You can serve your stir-fry over Cauliflower Rice (page 272).

2 tablespoons extra virgin olive oil, almond oil, or coconut oil
1¼ pounds skinless, boneless chicken breasts, cut into 1-inch pieces
2 cups broccoli florets
½ pound fresh mushrooms, sliced
4 scallions, cut into 1-inch pieces
3 tablespoons soy sauce
½ teaspoon ground ginger
1 teaspoon almond flour or coconut flour, dissolved in 2 tablespoons water
1 teaspoon sesame oil

In a large frying pan or wok, heat the oil over medium-high heat. Add the chicken cubes and stir-fry 3 minutes until the chicken becomes opaque. Remove with a slotted spoon and set aside.

Add the broccoli and stir-fry 1–2 minutes.

Add the mushrooms, scallions, soy sauce, ginger, and sesame oil. Stir-fry 2 more minutes.

Add the coconut or almond flour in water and the reserved chicken. Cook until heated through and the sauce has thickened.

You can serve this stir-fry over Cauliflower Rice.

Curried Chicken Salad in Lettuce Packages

Serves 4

A curried chicken salad is a great way to use up leftover whole roasted chicken or chicken breasts. You can buy an organic rotisserie chicken and use the meat to make the salad. Of course, you can poach or grill chicken breasts just for this purpose. It's a perfect lunch.

8 large Boston lettuce leaves
2 cups cooked chicken, diced
½ cup chopped celery
8 pitted black olives, chopped
2 tablespoons chopped scallions
10 cherry tomatoes, cut in half
2 tablespoons goji berries
¼ cup mayonnaise
½ teaspoon curry powder
¼ teaspoon sea salt
⅛ teaspoon freshly ground pepper

Bring a medium-size saucepan of water to a boil. Drop in the lettuce leaves. You are blanching the leaves. About a minute will do.

When wilted, drain in a colander under cold running water. Pat each leaf dry with paper towels. Your green wrap is ready.

In a medium-size bowl, combine the remaining ingredients and mix well.

Divide the chicken mixture into 8 equal portions. Place one portion in the middle of each lettuce leaf.

Fold the edges of each leaf toward the center to enclose the filling. Secure each package with a wooden toothpick.

Broiled Country Mustard Chicken

Serves 4

A no muss, no fuss recipe, this chicken has practically no prep time. You can prepare a salad and a vegetable as the chicken broils. It's a great weeknight meal when you don't have the time to tackle a more challenging one. And it delivers big flavor.

2 tablespoons coarse-grain Dijon mustard

2 tablespoons mayonnaise

2 scallions, thinly sliced

½ teaspoon dried basil

1 garlic clove, crushed through a press

¼ teaspoon freshly ground pepper

4 boneless chicken breast halves

Preheat the broiler. Place the shelf 6 inches from the heat.

In a small bowl, mix the mustard, mayonnaise, scallions, basil, garlic, and pepper.

Place the chicken pieces, skin side up, on a broiling pan.

Spread half the mustard mixture over the chicken.

Broil for 15–20 minutes, basting after 10 minutes.

Turn the chicken and spread the mustard mixture over the other side. Baste occasionally with the remaining sauce.

Let the Good Times Roll Spicy Pecan Chicken

Serves 4

New Orleans cuisine is hard to resist. Just as the city is a party that never ends, the food is renowned for its richness and zesty flavor. Louisiana with its Creole and Cajun food is one of the culinary capitals of the country. This quick recipe captures the zydeco spirit.

4 skinless, boneless chicken breast halves or thighs

¾ teaspoon dried thyme

½ teaspoon sea salt

¼ teaspoon freshly ground pepper

2 tablespoons extra virgin olive oil

1 tablespoon butter

½ cup coarsely chopped pecans

¼ cup sliced scallions

¼ cup dry white wine

¼–½ teaspoon Tabasco or other hot pepper sauce

Season the chicken with the thyme, salt, and pepper.

In a large frying pan, warm the olive oil over medium heat. Add the chicken and cook, turning once or twice, until the chicken is white throughout, 13–15 minutes.

Remove the chicken to a platter and cover with foil to keep warm.

Add the butter and pecans to the pan and cook, stirring, until the nuts are browned and fragrant, about 3 minutes.

Stir in the scallions and cook 30 seconds.

Add the wine and simmer 1 minute.

Stir in Tabasco to taste.

Pour the sauce over the chicken and serve.

A R C T I C   C H A R

Many people are nervous about cooking fish, but it's not a difficult skill to conquer. Arctic char is especially forgiving, because it is dense with omega-3s and hard to dry out. The recipes in this section are simple to make and just about fail proof. Once you get these down, you will be ready to tackle other fish recipes.

Arctic char has become very popular, because it is a very clean fish. Farm-grown char is safe to eat. Since you do not have to eat wild char, this option is reasonably priced. People love the flavor, which is more delicate than salmon.

Georgia's Pistachio-Crusted Arctic Char

Serves 6

Arctic char is a favorite omega-rich fish in our home. This recipe is my wife Georgia's favorite version. The sweet and crunchy pistachios combined with the richness of the fish make for a perfect marriage of flavors.

    1 cup shelled undyed pistachios
    ½ cup packed fresh basil leaves
    2 tablespoons minced shallots
    ¼ teaspoon sea salt
    ¼ teaspoon black pepper
    6½ tablespoons unsalted butter, softened
    6 6-ounce Arctic char fillets with skin, 1–1¼ inches thick
    ½ tablespoon olive oil

Preheat the oven to 400 degrees.

Coarsely chop the pistachios in a food processor. Add the basil, shallot, salt, pepper, and 6 tablespoons butter, and puree until the ingredients form a paste.

Remove any bones from the fish with tweezers and pat the fish dry.

Heat the olive oil and the remaining ½ tablespoon butter in a 12-inch nonstick skillet over moderately high heat until the foam subsides.

Place 3 fillets, skin side down, in the pan. Brown for 3–4 minutes. Transfer the fillets, skin sides down, to a lightly oiled 1-inch-deep baking pan.

Repeat with the remaining 3 fillets.

Divide the pistachio paste among the fillets and spread evenly in a ⅛-inch-thick layer on top of each.

Bake the fillets in the middle of the oven until just cooked through, 9–11 minutes.

Soy-Sesame Arctic Char

Serves 4

This seared char recipe has an Asian touch. Since it takes very little time to make, it is a perfect midweek recipe.

4 tablespoons soy sauce
1⅓ tablespoons honey
1 teaspoon toasted sesame oil
4 6-ounce Arctic char fillets with skin
coarse sea salt and freshly ground black pepper to taste

In a small bowl, stir together the soy sauce, honey, and sesame oil. Season the fish with salt and pepper and brush with half the sauce.

Heat a small cast-iron skillet or a nonstick skillet sprayed with olive oil over high heat. Sear the fish skin side up for 4 minutes.

Pour the remaining sauce over the fish and swirl around the pan. Carefully turn the fish, spoon the sauce over the top, and cook for 3 more minutes, until the fish is just cooked through. Serve immediately.

Baked Arctic Char with a Scallion Crust

Serves 2

This three-ingredient recipe is a perfect example of how easy it is to whip up an elegant main course that is as tasty as it is healthy.

4–6 scallions

1 tablespoon mayonnaise

2 6-ounce Arctic char fillets with skin

salt and pepper

Preheat the broiler. Line the rack of the broiler pan with foil.

Finely chop the scallions and stir in the mayonnaise.

Pat the fillets dry. Place the fillets, skin side down, on a broiler pan and season each fillet with salt and pepper. Spread the scallion mixture evenly over the tops of the fillets.

Broil 3–4 inches from the heat until the scallions are slightly charred and fish is just cooked through, about 8 minutes.

Garlic-Dill Baked Char

Serves 2–3

Here is another variation that takes no more than 25 minutes to make. The recipe doesn't require a lot of watching either. The fine flavor makes it seem more complicated than it is.

1 pound Arctic char fillet with skin

1 tablespoon extra virgin olive oil

3 tablespoons minced fresh dill

2 cloves garlic, minced

1 teaspoon sea salt

½ teaspoon pepper

1 lemon, quartered

Preheat the oven to 375 degrees.

Line a baking sheet with nonstick aluminum foil. Place the Arctic char on the baking sheet with the skin side facing down. Brush the flesh with olive oil.

In a small bowl, stir the dill, garlic, salt, and pepper together. Rub the flesh of the Arctic char with the mixture, distributed evenly.

Bake for 15–20 minutes until the fish flakes easily with a fork.

Cut into four pieces and serve with a lemon wedge.

Cajun Blackened Arctic Char

Serves 4–6

High flavor is the way to go with this dish. For the sake of convenience, this recipe calls for a ready-made mix of spices, which will do the trick.

Again, this is a simple entrée that will delight your taste buds.

2 tablespoons butter
2 tablespoons extra virgin olive oil
1 tablespoon Cajun spices
2 pounds Arctic char fillets, 1-inch thick with skin
1 lemon, plus lemon wedges for garnish

Melt the butter in a cast-iron or heavy-bottomed frying pan over medium-high heat and add the olive oil.

Add the Cajun spice and heat thoroughly.

Place the fillets in the pan. Squeeze the juice of the lemon into the pan.

Cook the fillets for about 5 minutes on each side.

Serve with the remaining lemon wedges and pan drippings.

M A I N C O U R S E

Meatless or Meaty* Chili

Serves 6–8

Chili is a great main course, but leftovers have many uses. You can serve a dollop on eggs, a burger or veggie burger, sausages, or chicken. It freezes well. You might want to try freezing the chili in individual portions so that you have some on hand when you do not feel like cooking or you need a quick bite.

        3 tablespoons extra virgin olive oil
        1 large onion, chopped
        1 red or green bell pepper, chopped
        2 garlic cloves, minced
        2 celery ribs, diced
        1 (14½-ounce) can Italian-style stewed tomatoes
        1 tablespoon balsamic or apple cider vinegar
        2 tablespoons chili powder
        2 teaspoons ground cumin
        ½ teaspoon dried basil
        8 ounces mushrooms, sliced
        2 medium zucchini, sliced
        2 large carrots, sliced
        2 (16-ounce) cans red kidney beans
        1½ teaspoons sea salt
        ¼ teaspoon cayenne
        ¼ cup chopped parsley
        1 small container sour cream (optional)
        1 avocado, sliced or cubed
        4 ounces grated cheddar, Monterey, or pepper jack cheese

In a large soup pot, heat the olive oil and cook the onion over medium heat, stirring occasionally, until softened, 2–3 minutes.

Add the bell pepper, garlic, and celery. Cook, stirring, until soft, 3–5 minutes.

Add the tomatoes, vinegar, chili powder, cumin, basil, mushrooms, zucchini, and carrots.

Cover, reduce heat to medium-low, and cook for 25 minutes.

Add the kidney beans with their liquid, salt, and cayenne to taste. Simmer, covered, for 10 minutes.

Sprinkle with parsley. Serve hot, with a dollop of sour cream, sliced avocado, and a sprinkling of the grated cheese of your choice.

*If you want beef, chicken, or turkey chili, brown a pound of grass-fed or organic chopped meat in the oil, stirring for about 5 minutes. Then add the onion and follow the rest of the recipe.

Variations on Guilt-Free Pizza

Serves 8

You do not have to go without pizza on my program. This outstanding recipe for a pizza crust made from cauliflower will allow you to make any kind of pie you want. I told you that cauliflower is a superfood!

1 head cauliflower, chopped into medium pieces
2 large eggs
½ cup shredded mozzarella cheese
2 tablespoons freshly grated Parmesan cheese
½ teaspoon dried oregano
½ teaspoon dried basil
½ teaspoon garlic powder
¼ teaspoon crushed red pepper flakes
¼ teaspoon sea salt

Preheat the oven to 425 degrees.

Line a baking sheet with a silicone baking mat or parchment paper.

Put the cauliflower into a food processor and pulse until finely ground. You should have about 2 or 3 cups.

Transfer the ground cauliflower into a microwave-safe bowl. Cover it loosely and cook in a microwave for 4–5 minutes, or until soft. Let it cool.

Using a clean dish towel or a piece of cheese cloth, drain the cauliflower by squeezing and twisting it. Remove as much water as possible.

Put the drained cauliflower into a large bowl. Stir in the rest of the ingredients.

Spread the mixture on the lined baking sheet into a 15-by-10-inch rectangle. Spray lightly with olive oil and bake for 12–15 minutes until golden brown.

Remove from the oven, put on your toppings, and return to the oven for 5–7 minutes.

Let the pizza cool for 2–3 minutes before slicing it.

Variations on Toppings

I don't have to tell you how to make a pizza with mozzarella, tomato sauce, and Italian seasoning. I thought I'd provide you with some adventurous combinations.

Roasted Vegetables and Goat Cheese

⅓ cup broccoli florets
½ red bell pepper, sliced
1¼ small red onions, sliced thin
3 tablespoons olive oil, divided
salt
1 cup mushrooms sliced
¼ cup pizza sauce or pesto
½ cup shredded mozzarella
1 ounce goat cheese, crumbled

Preheat the oven to 450 degrees.

Put the broccoli, bell peppers, and onions on a parchment-lined baking sheet. Drizzle with 2 tablespoons of olive oil and salt liberally. Bake for 8–10 minutes.

Sauté the mushrooms in a tablespoon of olive oil for 3–4 minutes.

Spread sauce on pizza crust, sprinkle with a layer of mozzarella. Then add the roasted vegetables, sautéed mushrooms, and crumbled goat cheese.

Put the pizza in the oven for 5–7 minutes. When the cheese is melted and bubbling, your pizza is ready.

Let rest for 2–3 minutes before slicing.

Gorgonzola and Caramelized Onion Pizza

If you like sweet and salty, this pizza is for you.

1 teaspoon extra virgin coconut oil
1 large yellow onion, thinly sliced
½ cup Gorgonzola cheese, crumbled
fresh thyme and rosemary to taste

Preheat the oven to 400 degrees.

While the crust is baking, melt the coconut oil in a skillet over medium heat and sauté the sliced onion.

After 20 minutes, during which you stir the onions occasionally, they should be soft and golden.

Arrange the onions and Gorgonzola on the crust and sprinkle with fresh thyme or rosemary.

Return the pizza to the oven and bake for 8–10 minutes, until the cheese has melted.

Fontina and Mushroom Pizza with a Fried Egg

Have you noticed how fried eggs are popping up in unexpected places? It is a definite trend. Why not pizza—especially one with mushrooms and fontina cheese?

2 tablespoons extra virgin olive oil
3 cloves garlic, minced
1 pound assorted mushrooms, sliced
1 tablespoon fresh thyme
salt
freshly ground black pepper
3 ounces fontina cheese, sliced
1 large egg
3 tablespoons chopped fresh parsley

Preheat the oven to 450 degrees.

In a large skillet, heat 1 tablespoon of olive oil on medium high. Add the garlic and cook about 1 minute.

Add the mushrooms and cook until golden brown, about 8 minutes. Add the thyme, salt, and pepper.

Lay half the fontina slices on the crust. Top the cheese with the mushrooms and then add another layer of cheese.

Bake in the oven until the cheese is bubbly.

While the pizza is baking, heat the remaining 1 tablespoon olive oil in a small, nonstick skillet over medium heat. Fry the egg for about 4 minutes, until the white is set and the yolk is still slightly runny. Season with salt and pepper.

When the pizza is out of the oven, place the egg in the center and sprinkle fresh parsley on the pizza.

French Green Lentils, Pears, and Shallot Salad with Arctic Char

Serves 4

This one-dish meal is textured and flavorful. Even better, you can get it on the table in just 30 minutes. It's great cold, so you will have tasty leftovers the next day.

    filtered water as needed
    1 cup French green lentils
    12-ounce Arctic char fillet with skin
    7 tablespoons cider vinegar, divided
    ½ cup diced shallots, divided
    1 large firm pear or Granny Smith apple, finely chopped
    1 tablespoon Dijon mustard
    ¼ teaspoon ground black pepper
    ⅛ teaspoon coarse sea salt
    4 scallions, very thinly sliced
    ¼ cup chopped fresh parsley

In a medium saucepan, bring 3 cups of water to a boil over high heat. Stir in the lentils, lower the heat, and simmer until they are tender, 18–20 minutes. Drain and set aside.

Put the Arctic char, 4 tablespoons vinegar, and ¼ cup shallots in the pan used for cooking the lentils. If necessary, fold the tail end of the char under to fit in the pan.

Add enough water to cover the fish. Bring the liquid to a simmer and lower the heat. Cover and cook until the fish is just opaque in the center, 5–6 minutes.

Remove the fish with a slotted spoon and transfer it to a plate.

Place the chopped pear or apple in the same pan on medium heat and cook until just warm, about 1 minute.

Add the remaining ¼ cup shallots and cooked lentils, cover, and cook, stirring occasionally until warmed, 4–5 minutes.

In a small bowl, whisk together the mustard, pepper, salt, and remaining 3 tablespoons vinegar. Pour the dressing over the lentils, add the scallions and parsley, and toss to combine.

Flake the fish away from the skin and serve over lentils.

CAULIFLOWER

Cauliflower is another trendy food today. People are concerned about cutting down their carbohydrate intake, and cauliflower saves the day. When I recommend not eating anything white, cauliflower is not on that list. It is a superfood you should be eating more of.

Mediterranean Oven-Roasted Cauliflower

Serves 4

Garlic, olive oil, and lemon juice taste great on just about anything—and cauliflower is no exception.

    1 medium head of cauliflower, broken up into 5–6 cups florets, about
        1½ inches in diameter
    ¼ cup extra virgin olive oil
    1 tablespoon sliced garlic
    2 tablespoons lemon juice
    1 teaspoon sea salt
    ½ teaspoon black pepper
    2 tablespoons grated Parmesan cheese
    chopped parsley or chives, for garnish

Preheat the oven to 500 degrees.

Place the cauliflower florets in a large roasting pan. Drizzle the olive oil over the cauliflower, and season with the garlic, lemon juice, salt, and pepper.

Place the roasting pan in the oven for 15 minutes, stirring occasionally.

Remove the pan from the oven and sprinkle with the Parmesan cheese. Garnish with chopped parsley or chives and serve immediately.

Brown Butter Drizzled Cauliflower Steaks with Pumpkin Seeds and Lime

Serves 4

Cauliflower steaks are in! They look great on a dish. This is a sophisticated way to serve up this superfood.

2 tablespoons extra virgin olive oil, divided
1 large head cauliflower
coarse sea salt
freshly ground pepper
2 tablespoons unsalted butter
¼ cup raw shelled pumpkin seeds
½ teaspoon crushed red pepper flakes
¼ cup chopped fresh cilantro
1 tablespoon fresh lime juice

Preheat the oven to 450 degrees.

Coat a large rimmed baking sheet with 1 tablespoon oil.

Trim the cauliflower stalk and place the head stalk side down on a cutting board. Slice the cauliflower lengthwise into ½-inch slices.

Arrange the cauliflower slices and any stray pieces in a single layer on the prepared baking sheet. Drizzle with 1 tablespoon olive oil and season with salt and pepper.

Roast until the underside is deeply browned, 20–25 minutes.

Turn the cauliflower over, season with additional salt and pepper, and continue to roast until the other side is dark brown and crisp, 15–20 minutes longer.

While the cauliflower is browning, melt the butter in a small skillet over medium heat. Add the pumpkin seeds, bring to a simmer, and cook. Swirl the pan occasionally, until the pumpkin seeds are toasted and butter is browned and smells nutty, 6–8 minutes.

Remove from the heat and add the red pepper flakes. Let the pumpkin seeds cool 10 minutes.

Add the chopped cilantro and lime juice. Season with salt and pepper.

Arrange the cauliflower on a serving platter and drizzle with dressing.

Serve topped with fresh cilantro leaves.

Lemon Parsley Roasted Cauliflower

Serves 4

Another classic, this recipe is one I never get tired of. If you have any left-overs, you can always eat the cauliflower cold as a snack, toss it into a salad, or use it as a crudité.

2-pound head of cauliflower, cut into florets, including tender leaves
6 tablespoons extra virgin olive oil, divided
coarse sea salt
freshly ground pepper
1 cup fresh flat-leaf parsley leaves
2 tablespoons fresh lemon juice
½ teaspoon finely grated lemon zest

Preheat the oven to 425 degrees.
Toss the cauliflower and 4 tablespoons of the olive oil on a rimmed baking sheet. Season with salt and pepper.
Roast, tossing occasionally, until golden brown and tender, 25–30 minutes.
While the cauliflower is roasting, pulse the parsley, lemon juice, and remaining 2 tablespoons of olive oil in a food processor until very finely chopped. Season with salt and pepper to taste.
When the cauliflower is ready, toss the florets with the lemon-parsley mixture and top with lemon zest.

I Can't Believe It's Not Mashed Potatoes

Serves 4

Low-carb mashed potatoes—what could be better? This is an especially rich version, because on the Triple A Diet you can have sour cream.

1 head cauliflower, cut into 6–7 cups of florets
1 cup water
3 tablespoons milk
1 tablespoon butter
2 tablespoons sour cream
¼ teaspoon sea salt
2 cloves minced garlic
freshly ground black pepper

Separate the cauliflower into florets and chop the core finely.

Bring the water to a simmer in a pot, then add the cauliflower. Cover and turn the heat to medium. Cook the cauliflower for 12–15 minutes or until very tender.

Drain and discard the water. Add the milk, butter, sour cream, salt, garlic, and pepper and process in a food processer or mash with a masher until the cauliflower looks like mashed potatoes.

Variation on Mashed Cauliflower

Serves 4

If you want to keep the dairy products out of your mashed cauliflower, this recipe is an easy way to do it.

1 medium head cauliflower, trimmed and cut into 6–7 cups of florets
1 tablespoon extra virgin olive oil
2 cloves minced garlic
fine sea salt and ground black pepper to taste

Bring a large pot of salted water to a boil.

Add the cauliflower and cook until very tender, about 10 minutes.

Reserve ¼ cup of the cooking liquid and then drain the cauliflower well. Transfer the cauliflower to a food processor. Add the oil, garlic, and reserved water, 1 tablespoon at a time. Puree until smooth. Or you can mash cauliflower with a potato masher.

Season with salt and pepper and serve.

Centerpiece Cauliflower

Serves 4–6 as a side dish, 2 as a main course

Roasting time: 1–2 hours

A striking way to serve cauliflower is to roast the entire head until it turns golden brown and to serve it whole. You can drizzle olive oil over the cauliflower, season it with salt and pepper, and roast it for about an hour. I prefer a more elaborate method, because the cauliflower is more tender. Once you get the technique down, you can sauce the roasted cauliflower any way you would like to.

To Roast the Cauliflower

> 1 large cauliflower
> olive oil
> sea salt

Preheat the oven to 375 degrees.

Place a heavy, oven-proof skillet or a baking sheet in the warming oven. Put a small pan of hot water on the floor of the oven, to create steam.

Prepare the cauliflower for roasting by breaking off the outer leaves from the cauliflower. Cut off the bottom of the stem. Use the tip of a knife to cut out the hard core. Leave the main stem intact and make sure not to cut through any of the florets.

Rinse the cauliflower. Place on a work surface, core side up. Drizzle with olive oil and use your hands to rub over the cauliflower until evenly coated. Sprinkle with salt.

Place the cauliflower on the hot pan in the oven, core side down, and cook until very tender all the way through when pierced with a knife, at least 1 hour or up to 2 hours.

During the cooking, baste 2 or 3 times with more olive oil.

When the cauliflower is tender, place it under the broiler for a short time until the surface is golden brown.

A Sauce Option

> ⅓ cup blanched (skinless) almonds
> 2 garlic cloves, peeled
> 2 tablespoons unsalted butter
> ½ cup extra virgin olive oil
> 2 teaspoons white vinegar
> ½ cup coarsely chopped fresh herbs such as parsley, mint, tarragon, cilantro, or a combination
> ¼ to 1 teaspoon red pepper flakes
> salt and ground black pepper

In a small frying pan, toast the almonds over low heat until they are golden, shaking often. Let cool.

In a food processor, combine the almonds, garlic, and butter and pulse until smooth. Add the oil, then vinegar. Then mix in the herbs and red pepper flakes, if using. Season to taste with salt and pepper. Set aside.

Serve the cauliflower in the skillet or from a serving plate. Pour some sauce over the head. When serving, cut the cauliflower into wedges and spoon the remaining sauce around each wedge.

"Kill Your Carb Craving" Cauliflower Rice Basic Recipe

Serves 8

One of the latest food trends is to substitute cauliflower rice for white rice. If you want to avoid simple carbs yet have a bed of something white under your chili or want a starchy side dish, cauliflower rice will let you have it both ways.

Creating the "Rice"

All you need is a head of cauliflower.

After removing the leaves, cut the cauliflower into quarters and cut out the core. Go on to cut each quarter in a few chunks.

Working with half the cauliflower at a time, process the florets for about 30 seconds until the cauliflower looks like fine rice or couscous.

If you don't have a food processor, you can grate the cauliflower on the coarse side of a grater.

You can store the "rice" in the refrigerator for 3 days. It will last in the freezer in freezer-locked plastic bags for up to 3 months. It's a good idea to make a batch so that you have the "rice" on hand. You can defrost the cauliflower rice in a microwave and get cooking.

How to Cook the Rice

You have a choice of how to prepare your rice: roasting, microwaving, or stir-frying.

Roasting

Preheat the oven to 425 degrees.

Toss the rice in a little extra virgin olive oil.

Cover a baking sheet with parchment paper and put the cauliflower rice on the sheet, spread out evenly into a thin layer.

Put the baking sheet into the oven. After 6 minutes, stir the rice and spread it out thin again. Roast for 6 more minutes.

Microwaving

Put the cauliflower rice in a microwave-proof bowl and cover with plastic wrap. Microwave on high for 3 minutes. If you are using the rice straight from the freezer, cook for 4 minutes on high, mixing the rice halfway through cooking.

Stir-Frying

Simply stir-fry the cauliflower rice in a little extra virgin olive oil for 5 minutes.

Once you have your cauliflower rice, you can use it as you would cooked rice. Check online to explore all the possibilities.

Cauliflower Fried Rice

Serves 6

This recipe fooled me! I thought I was cheating when Georgia served it to me, but this version of "fried rice" is on the program. Indulge! You'll love it.

2 tablespoons extra virgin olive oil

1 medium onion, diced

2 garlic cloves, minced

1 tablespoon toasted sesame oil

¼ cup low-sodium soy sauce

2 carrots, sliced

2 cups snow peas

3 stalks celery, sliced

4–6 cups cooked cauliflower rice

2 eggs, beaten

3 scallions, thinly sliced

¼ cup cashews

Heat the olive oil in a wok or large frying pan over medium-high heat.

Add the onion and cook for 5 minutes. Then add the garlic and cook for another minute.

Stir in the toasted sesame oil and soy sauce.

Raise the heat to high. Add the carrots, snow peas, and celery and cook for about 5 minutes. Continue to toss.

Add the cooked cauliflower rice and toss until warm.

Add the eggs and toss until they are stringy.

Top with scallions and cashews.

You can add shrimp, chicken, scallions, or beef to this fried rice to make it a main course.

SALADS

With all the salad bars available today, I did not think that recipes for mixed green salads would enlighten you. Instead, I have tried to broaden your horizons with a few new recipes.

Quinoa: The Perfect "Grain" as a Blank Canvas

You might be tired of hearing about quinoa or you might never have tried it on principle. Quinoa is a complete protein. It contains all of the essential amino acids. It also passes for a very starchy grain. If you have not developed a taste for it already, give it a try. It will grow on you. It's all a matter of what you do with it.

Vegetable Medley Quinoa

(Week 4)

Serves 4

Quinoa is so nutritious and versatile—I can't get enough of it. Quinoa is a satisfying substitute for rice and pasta. When you reach Week 4 on the program, you might want to keep some cooked quinoa in your refrigerator all the time. All you have to do is chop up some vegetables and toss them with quinoa and salad dressing.

Try this basic recipe, and then create your own delicious combinations of your favorite vegetables. Be creative—you can use any kind of raw, sautéed, or roasted vegetables. Cooked quinoa is a great second act for leftover vegetables. The recipe below gives you a combination I enjoy, but you can use whatever vegetables you like. I even eat leftovers with my eggs in the morning. There is no wrong time of day to eat quinoa.

4 ribs celery, chopped

2 carrots, chopped

1 medium red onion, chopped

1 tablespoon extra virgin olive oil (2 tablespoons if you sauté the vegetables)

1 cup uncooked quinoa

2 cups filtered water or low-sodium vegetable stock

4 cloves garlic, peeled

sea salt and pepper to taste

parsley or cilantro for garnish

Set aside if leaving raw. For less crunch, sauté with 1 tablespoon olive oil in a medium saucepan over medium-low heat until tender, about 5 minutes.

Rinse the uncooked quinoa in a fine strainer.

Add the quinoa to a pot along with 2 cups of liquid.

Add the peeled garlic cloves, 1 tablespoon olive oil, salt, and pepper, and bring the liquid to a boil.

Reduce the heat to low and let simmer for 15 minutes or until all the liquid is absorbed by quinoa.

Mix in the vegetables.

Garnish with the parsley or cilantro.

Variations: Add chopped nuts and/or ½ cup cubed or shaved cheese—goat, feta, mozzarella, cheddar, Swiss, Manchego, shaved Parmesan, or Romano.

Red Quinoa Salad with a Crunch Factor

Serves 4 (Week 4)

You can use white quinoa in this salad, but the red quinoa with shaved cauliflower looks very colorful on the plate. This is a round-the-clock salad that works any time of day.

½ cup red quinoa

½ head cauliflower, coarsely grated

½ cup finely chopped parsley (save leaves for garnish)

¼ cup roughly chopped pitted Kalamata olives

⅓ cup extra virgin olive oil

⅓ cup toasted, chopped walnuts

2 tablespoons lemon juice

1 teaspoon lemon zest

½ teaspoon ground cumin

coarse sea salt and freshly ground black pepper

Bring a large pot of salted water to a boil.

Add the quinoa and simmer until fully cooked, about 15 minutes. Drain and return the quinoa to the pot. Cover with a lid and let it sit for 5 additional minutes. Fluff the quinoa with a fork and transfer to a large bowl or sheet pan to cool.

Combine the cooled quinoa and the remaining ingredients in a large bowl. Season with salt, pepper, and more lemon juice if desired. Transfer the salad to a large serving bowl or platter and garnish with parsley.

Serve cold or at room temperature.

Green Bean Salad with Red Quinoa

Serves 4

You can use quinoa as a condiment rather than the base of a dish. This simple salad is colorful and has a lot going on with crunch. This salad is a great way to use leftover quinoa.

1 pound green beans, trimmed

3–4 tablespoons chopped red onion

½ cup chopped toasted almonds

1 Serrano or Thai chili pepper, minced—use more if you like it hot. If you don't have hot peppers available, a splash of Sriracha to taste will work.

⅓ cup cilantro, chopped

2 tablespoons chives, minced

3 tablespoons fresh lime juice

Celtic Sea Salt to taste

⅓ cup extra virgin olive oil

1¼ cups cooked red quinoa

2 hard-boiled eggs, finely chopped

Fill a medium saucepan with water and bring to a boil. Add salt and green beans.

Boil 4–5 minutes until the beans are crisply tender.

While the beans are cooking, soak the onion in cold water for 5 minutes. Soaking red onions in water eliminates their harsh bite.

Drain the beans and transfer them to a bowl of cold water to stop them from cooking more. Drain again. Wrap the beans in a kitchen towel to absorb water.

Combine the green beans, onion, almonds, chili, cilantro, and chives in a salad bowl.

Make a lime dressing by combining the lime juice, salt, and olive oil in a small covered jar and shake. If you don't have a jar, use a small bowl and whisk the ingredients together.

Toss the dressing with the beans.

Add the cooked quinoa and toss again.

Sprinkle chopped egg on top and serve.

Cucumber and Celery Refresher

Serves 4

You can make this salad in a flash as a perfect side dish. The recipe calls for parsley and mint, but you can use any herb combination you would like. Dill, tarragon, savory, and oregano all would work well.

6 celery stalks, thinly sliced
1 seedless cucumber, peeled and thinly sliced
⅓ cup coarsely chopped fresh flat-leaf parsley
¼ cup coarsely chopped fresh mint
3 tablespoons extra virgin olive oil
coarse salt and freshly ground black pepper

Toss the celery, cucumber, parsley, mint, and oil together in a bowl. Season with salt and pepper.

Superfood Special: Kale, Avocado, and Olive Salad

Serves 1–2

If you find raw kale tough and bitter, the preparation technique used in this recipe to prepare the dark green leaves transforms this superfood. Give it a try!

1 head kale
¼ teaspoon salt
1 lemon, squeezed
½ avocado, mashed
½ carrot, chopped
¼ cup black olives, pitted and chopped
4 tablespoons chopped fresh herbs of your choice
¼ cup raw cashews
¼ cup sprouts (optional)

Remove the kale from the thick stems. Place the leaves in a large bowl and salt the leaves.

Massage the leaves. The salt will wilt the kale.

Do the same with the lemon juice.

Then massage the leaves with the avocado until it's well incorporated.

Taste. You might need more lemon juice or salt.

Cut the kale into strips and place it in a serving bowl.

Add the rest of the ingredients and toss to combine.

S N A C K S

You will not go hungry on the Triple A Diet. Two snacks a day are built into the meal plans. I am not talking about junk food. Instead of potato chips, think kale chips. There are so many things you can eat that will boost your energy instead of causing you to burn and crash. This section has a few of my favorites to get you started on eating for balance.

Crispy Roasted Vegetables

Serves as many as you make

Crunchy roasted vegetables are a delicious side dish and snack. You can throw leftovers into cooked quinoa, cauliflower rice, or an omelet. I eat bowls of them during the day. I love Brussels sprouts, broccoli, carrots, parsnips, eggplant, cauliflower, green beans, halved cherry or grape tomatoes, red onions, and butternut squash, just to name a few vegetables done this way. If you roast kale, you have kale chips! Yum. Sometimes I mix the vegetables for a colorful snack. You can combine roasted vegetables with quinoa for a balanced meal. Experiment with seasoning. I like to use cumin on carrots or basil and garlic with the tomatoes.

Preheat the oven to 350 degrees.

Prepare the vegetables as if you were going to steam them—in bite-sized pieces.

Put the vegetables in a plastic bag, add a little extra virgin olive oil, and shake to coat. Do not use too much oil.

Line a baking sheet with parchment paper to save on cleanup time.

Spread vegetables in a single layer on a baking sheet. Season well with sea salt.

Bake for 25–45 minutes—depending on how crisp you want your veggies to be and the size of the pieces. Smaller pieces cook more quickly.

Tropical Kale Chips

Serves 4–6

My family is addicted to this healthy snack. If you crave chips, this simple recipe will satisfy. The flavor of coconut makes these chips especially delicious—and healthier. Enjoy!

 1 bunch kale
 ¼ cup organic virgin coconut oil
 sea salt to taste

Cut the thick stem from each kale leaf. Place a few leaves on top of each other, roll into a cigar shape, and slice. Open and cut the slices in half or thirds, depending on how long they are.

 Melt the coconut oil in a frying pan large enough to hold all the pieces of kale. Stir to coat the kale with coconut oil. Salt liberally. Stir for 5–10 minutes. The color will darken and the leaves will get soft. Just keep stirring and they will get hard and crisp and ready to eat.

Grace's Blast-Off Bars

Serves 10

Cooling time: 90 minutes

My daughter, Grace, is known for her love of travel, exploration, and the great outdoors. She also has an amazing energy and spirit, and these grainless energy bars mirror this. We love it when she makes them for the whole family.

 1 cup raw almonds
 10 pitted Medjool dates
 ¼ cup unsweetened shredded coconut, plus 1 tablespoon for topping
 2 tablespoons chia seeds
 1 teaspoon filtered water
 ½ cup cashew butter
 2 tablespoons extra virgin coconut oil
 ¼ cup honey
 ¼ cup goji berries

Place the almonds, dates, shredded coconut, chia seeds, and water in a food processor.

Pulse until the ingredients form a meal, sandy but not fine.

Transfer the mixture into a large bowl.

In a small saucepan, combine the cashew butter and coconut oil over medium heat until smooth, about 2–3 minutes.

Pour the warm mixture over the meal.

Add the honey and goji berries and mix together.

Transfer the mixture to an 8-by-8-inch square baking dish lined with wax paper or parchment paper.

Spread the mixture evenly and top with shredded coconut.

Place in the freezer for 90 minutes before removing and cutting the bars.

Yummy Oat Bars

(Week 4)

Serves 12

Cooling time: 3 hours

These yummy bars contain oats, which is why you have to wait until Week 4 to enjoy them.

2 cups oats

¼ cup shelled salted pistachios, chopped

3 tablespoons flaxseeds

⅓ cup organic honey

2 teaspoons pure vanilla extract

2 tablespoons extra virgin coconut oil

2½ tablespoons almond butter

¼ cup dried goji berries

Preheat the oven to 350 degrees.

Line a large baking sheet with parchment paper. Arrange the oats in a single layer and bake for 10–15 minutes. Make sure to check them, so they don't burn. When they are golden brown, take them out and set the baking sheet aside to cool.

Transfer the oats to a large bowl. Add the chopped pistachios and flaxseeds and toss well.

In a small saucepan, combine the honey, vanilla extract, and coconut oil. Cook over medium-low heat, stirring constantly until the coconut oil has melted.

Whisk in the almond butter and continue cooking for 1–2 minutes.

Remove the pan from the heat and add the goji berries.

Pour the mixture over the oats and mix well with a wooden spoon until they are evenly coated.

Use olive oil cooking spray to coat an 11-by-7-inch nonstick baking pan. Transfer the oat mixture into the pan. Press the mixture to make it even. The more you press, the better the bars will stick together. Refrigerate the pan until the oat mixture is firm, at least 2 hours.

Cut into 12 bars and remove with a spatula. Keep the bars refrigerated.

Peak Energy Trail Mix

Serves 6–8

Soaking and overnight dehydration time (optional): 4–6 hours

You should keep a small bag of this quick pick-me-up snack with you as you race through your day. Not only is it energizing, but it will also chase away hunger pangs—the perfect solution for carb cravings.

It is a good idea to sprout the sunflower seeds for optimum nutrition, but if you are pressed for time, you can skip it.

   1 cup raw sunflower seeds, preferably soaked for 4–6 hours and
      dehydrated overnight
   2 tablespoons hemp seeds
   2 tablespoons cacao nibs
   2 tablespoons goji berries
   1 teaspoon cinnamon
   ¼ teaspoon sea salt
   1 tablespoon raw honey
   2 tablespoons shredded coconut

In a large bowl, toss together the sunflower seeds, hemp seeds, cacao nibs, goji berries, cinnamon, and salt. Mix well.

Add the honey and toss well so that the ingredients are evenly coated.

Toss coconut into the mix.

Store in a covered container.

Goji Almond Butter Truffles

Serves 12

Soaking time: 1 hour

These buttery snacks go down smoothly despite their chunky consistency. They are full of protein, Vitamin E, antioxidants, and a host of other nutrients. They are a treat that packs a nutritional punch.

2 cups raw almonds
¼ cup goji berries, soaked in 1 cup of water for 1 hour
¼ cup hemp seeds
¼ cup honey
½ cup filtered water

Blend all the ingredients in a food processor for 2–5 minutes. Scrape the sides down. You are aiming for a dough-like consistency.

Roll the dough into bite-size truffles.

You can refrigerate these truffles in an airtight glass container for 4 days.

Coconut Bliss Balls

Serves 12

A perfect snack or dessert, these coconut balls have an irresistible flavor. They are so delicious, it's hard to believe they are so low in sugar! When you have a sweet craving, here is the answer.

1 cup raw cashews
1 cup dried coconut
2 tablespoons goji berries
1 pinch sea salt
1 lemon, juiced
rind of 2 lemons
⅓ cup maple syrup
1 tablespoon vanilla extract

Blend the cashews, coconut, 1 tablespoon of goji berries, and salt into a fine flour.

With the processor turned on, add the lemon juice, lemon rind, maple syrup, and vanilla, and blend to the consistency of dough.

Add the remaining goji berries for crunch and blend for another minute.

Roll the mixture into balls slightly larger than a quarter. Cool on a plate in the refrigerator until firm, about 15 minutes.

Afterword

Balance Is Everything

Now you have a step-by-step plan for fighting health-destroying inflammation. You are on the road to balance. My patients tell me they have benefited from having a map to follow. They say that the Curatola Care Program has dramatically improved their health—and not only their oral health, but their sense of well-being as well. They feel as if they have rebooted their bodies. I hope your experience has been the same.

Now that you have read *The Mouth⇔Body Connection*, I want to keep you in the loop as I do for my patients. My website features my blogs, coverage of up-to-the-minute breakthroughs in research, recipes, supplement information, video clips of yoga, meditation techniques, and workouts, and a wealth of wellness information. Revitin® Prebiotic Toothpaste is available on the website.

Acknowledgments

It is with deep appreciation that I acknowledge the following people for their contributions to this book:

Diane Reverand, my coauthor, brought her experience and exceptional literary career to this collaboration, which made it possible for me not only to make this book a reality, but to offer practical, understandable, and actionable information. Thank you to family friend Melody Weir, for bringing Diane and me together!

I offer my gratitude to my literary agent, David Vigliano, whose brilliant creative mind also helped make this book a reality by effectively representing and communicating its value to the publishing community.

Thanks to Kate Hartson, my editor at Hachette Center Street, whose tireless work, support, and fresh ideas have helped make this book a compelling contribution to the world of health and wellness, and her indefatigable assistant, Grace Tweedy. Thanks also to the entire team at Hachette, including Andrea Glickson and her marketing department.

I don't know how I would get through a day without the help of the terrific members of my staff. Thank you Rubina Montapert, our practice coordinator, who keeps wheels turning smoothly, Marta Komar and Jose Rojas, my stellar dental assistants, and Cortney Annese, my incomparable dental hygienist.

Special thanks go to my colleagues and special friends, Dr. Jack Tips, a brilliant naturopathic doctor, and Dr. Shayne Morris, a visionary molecular biologist, for their contributions to the cellular nutrition and dietary supplements included in this book. A note of gratitude goes to one of my most generous and loving friends, Sarica Cernhous, a whole-food nutritionist and natural lifestyle consultant, for her contributions on lacto-fermented foods, and the Weston A. Price diet. Adam Zickerman, a friend of Diane's and mine, the founder of InForm Fitness, applied his passion and considerable experience to design the workouts for the program.

The completion of this book has had the support of many friends and doctors in the health care community, but a special thanks to my older brother, Dr. Dominick Curatola, a true doctor, mentor, and brilliant cardiologist; my younger sister and fellow dentist, Dr. LuAnne Curatola; my brother-in-law and dentist, Dr. Joseph Zagami; and many dear friends, including, Dr. Dan Pompa, Dr. Isaac Jones, Dr. Guido Sarnachiaro, Dr. Josh Wagner, Dr. Greg Mongeon, Dr. Scott Werner, Dr. Jay Davidson, Dr. Josh Axe, Dr. Mehmet Oz, Dr. Jeffrey Bland, Dr. Tierona LowDog, and Dr. Joe Mercola. Thank you all for listening to what I had to say and supporting me for many years.

Selected Sources

p. 2: Gum disease in-depth report. www.nytimes.com /health/guides/disease/periodontitis/print.html.

p. 15: Countless studies have been done on the relationship between the oral microbiome and systemic inflammation and disease. Here are just a few:

Hajishengallis, George. Periodontitis: From microbial immune subversion to systemic inflammation. *Nature Reviews Immunology.* 2015, 15: 30–44, doi:10.1038/nri3785.

Li, Xiaojing, Kristen M. Kollveit, Leif Tronstad, and Ingar Olsen. Systemic diseases caused by oral infection. *Clinical Microbiology Reviews.* Oct 2000, 13(4): 547–58.

Otomo-Corgel, Joan. The most important perio-systemic facts. http://www.rdhmag.com/articlesprint/volumn-33/issue-12 /features/the-most-important-perio-systemic-facts.html.

Paquette, David W. The periodontal infection–systemic disease link: A review of truth or myth. *Journal of the International Academy of Periodontology.* Aug 2002, 4(3): 101–9.

Wade, William G. The oral microbiome in health and disease. *Pharmacological Research.* 2013, 69: 137–43.

p. 28: Keller, Amelie, Jeanett F. Rohde, Keil Raymond, and Berit L. Heitmann. Association between periodontal disease and overweight and obesity: A systemic review. *Journal of Periodontology.* June 2015, 86(6): 766–76, doi:10.1902/jop.2015.140589.

p. 29: Goodson, J. M., D. Groppo, S. Halem, and E. Carpino. Is obesity an oral bacterial disease? *Journal of Dental Research.* June 2009, 88(6): 519–23, doi:10.1177/0022034509338353.

p. 32: Kostic, A. D., D. Gevers, C. S. Pedamallu, M. Michaud, F. Duke, A. M. Earl, A. I. Ojesina, et al. Genomic analysis identifies association of fusobacterium with colorectal carcinoma. *Genome Research.* Oct 18, 2011, 22(2): 292–98, doi:10.1101/gr.126573.111.

p. 36: Hooper, Lora, and Jeff Gordon. Commensal host-bacterial relationships in the gut. *Science.* May 11, 2001, 292(5519): 1115–18.

p. 36: Neuroinflammation Working Group, Haruhiko Akiyama, Steven Barger, Scott Barnum, Bonnie Bradt, et al. Inflammation and Alzheimer's disease. *Neurobiology of Aging.* May-Jun 2000, 21(3): 383–421.

p. 37: Li, Xiaojing, Kristin M. Kolltveit, Leif Tronstad, and Ingar Olsen. Systemic diseases caused by oral infection. *Clinical Microbiology Reviews.* Oct 2000, 13(4): 547–58.

p. 40: Kim, Jemin, and Salomon Amar. Periodontal disease and systemic conditions: A bidirectional relationship. *Odontology.* Sep 2006, 94(1): 10–21. doi: 10.1007/s10266-006 -0060-6.

Michaud, Dominique S., Kaumudi Joshipura, Edward Giovannucci, and Charles S. Fuchs. A prospective study of periodontal disease and pancreatic cancer in US male health professionals. *Journal of the National Cancer Institute.* January 17, 2007.

p. 40: Michaud, D. S., Y. Liu, M. Meyer, E. Giovannucci, and K. Joshipura. Periodontal disease, tooth loss, and cancer risk in male health professionals: A prospective cohort study. *Lancet Oncology.* Jun 2008 (epub: May 5, 2008), 9(6):550–58, doi: 10.1016/S1470-2045(08)70106-2.

p. 40: Bui, T. C., C. M. Markham, M. W. Ross, and P. D. Mullen. Examining the association between oral health and oral HPV infection. *Cancer Prevention Research.* Sep 2013, 6(9): 917–24. doi:10.1158/1940-6207.

p. 46: Hooper, Lora, and Jeff Gordon. Commensal host-bacterial relationships in the gut. *Science.* May 11, 2001, 292(5519): 1115–18.

Lederberg, J. Infectious history. *Science.* Apr 14, 2000, 288(5464): 287–93.

p. 60: Kobylewski, S., and M. F. Jacobson. Toxicology of food dyes. *International Journal of Occupational and Environmental Health.* Jul-Sep 2012, 18(3): 220–46, doi:10.1179/10773525 12Z.00000000034.

p. 74:   https://www.ewg.org/skindeep/ingredient/718373 /DIETHANOLAMINE/.

p. 78: Columbia University College of Dentistry. Fluoride treatments and supplements. http://www.colgate.com/en/us /oc/oral-health/basics/fluoride/article/flouride-treatments -and-supplements.

p. 75: Choi, Anna L., Guifan Sun, Ying Zhang, and Philippe Grandjean. Developmental fluoride neurotoxicity: A systematic review and meta-analysis. *Environmental Health Perspectives.* Oct 2012 (online: Jul 20, 2012), 120(10): 1362–68, doi: 10.1289/ehp.1104912.

Iheozor-Ejiofor, Zipporah, Helen V. Worthington, Tanya Walsh, Lucy O'Malley, Jan E. Clarkson, Richard Macey, Rahul Alam, Peter Tugwell, Vivian Welch, and Anne-Marie Glenny. Water fluoridation for the prevention of dental caries. *Cochrane Database of Systematic Reviews.* 2015, Issue 6, Art. No. CD010856, doi:10.1002/14651858.CD010856.pub2.

Lu, Y., Z. R. Sun, L. N. Wu, X. Wang, W. Lu, and S. S. Liub. Effect of high-fluoride water on intelligence in children: Tianjin, China. *Fluoride.* 2000, 33(2): 74–78.

Malin, Ashley J., and Christine Till. Exposure to fluoridated water and attention deficit hyperactivity disorder prevalence among children and adolescents in the United States: An ecological association. *Environmental Health.* 2015, 14(17), doi:10.1186/s12940-015-0003-1.

Peckham, S., D. Lowery, and S. Spencer. Are fluoride levels in drinking water associated with hypothyroidism prevalence in England? A large observational study of GP practice data and fluoride levels in drinking water. *Journal of Epidemiology & Community Health*. doi:10.1136.

p. 76: Rule, K. L., V. R. Ebbett, and P. J. Vikesland. Formation of chloroform and chlorinated organics by free-chlorine-mediated oxidation of triclosan. *Environmental Science & Technology*. 2005, 39(9): 3176–85.

p. 77: Pharmaceuticals, hormones, and other organic wastewater contaminants in U.S. streams. Jun 2002. USGS Fact Sheet FS-027-02 (PDF [372k]).

p. 78: Kobylewski, S., and, M. F. Jacobson. Toxicology of food dyes. Jul-Sep 2012, 18(3): 220–46, doi:10.1179/10773525 12Z.00000000034.

p. 84: Curatola, Gerald P. Oral microbiome homeostasis: The new frontier in oral care therapies. *Symbiosis. Journal of Dentistry, Oral Disorders & Therapy*. Dec 22, 2013, 1(1): 3, doi:http://dx.doi.org/10.15226/jdodt.2013.00105.

Daniels, Anita H., and Steven R. Jefferies. Analysis of capacity of novel, antioxidant toothpaste to reduce gingival inflammation in pilot, small-population. Clinical study: Comparison to levels of gingival inflammation reduction reported in historical control and therapeutic toothbrushing studies. Independent study.

Pameijer, C. H., N. Grande, G. Plotino, A. Butti, A. Lerda, and V. Pasquali. An evaluation of the effectiveness of an experimental oral therapy paste (Revitin® with NuPath® Bioactives) on oral soft tissue health. Independent study.

Understanding risk assessment for mercury from dental amalgam. https://iaomt.org/understanding-risk-assessment-mercury-dental-amalgam/.

p. 100: IAOMT. The scientific case against amalgam. http://www.fda.gov/ohrms/dockets/dockets/06n0352/06N-0352-EC22-Attach-28.pdf.

p. 100: Evaluation of risks associated with mercury vapor from dental amalgam. Prepared by the Subcommittee on Risk Assessment Committee to Coordinate Environmental Health and Related Programs. Nov 7, 1991 (rev. Aug 28, 1992). https://health.gov/environment/amalgam1/appendixiii.htm.

Gebel, T., and H. Dunkelberg. Influence of chewing gum consumption and dental contact of amalgam fillings to different metal restorations on urine mercury content. *Zentralblatt für Hygiene und Umweltmedizin [International Journal of Hygiene and Environmental Health].* Nov 1996, 199(1): 69–75.

Sällsten, G., J. Thorén, L. Barregård, A. Schütz, and G. Skarping. Long-term use of nicotine chewing gum and mercury exposure from dental amalgam fillings. *Journal of Dental Research.* Jan 1996, 75(1): 594–98.

p. 131: Rennard, B. O., R. F. Ertl, G. L. Gossman, R. A. Robbins, and S. I. Rennard. Chicken soup inhibits neutrophil chemotaxis in vitro. *Chest.* Oct 2000, 118(4): 1150–57.

p. 133: Oh, Kyungwon, Frank B. Hu, Meir J. Stampfer, and Walter C. Willett. Dietary fat intake and risk of coronary heart disease in women: 20 years of follow-up of the Nurses' Health Study. *American Journal of Epidemiology.* 2005, 161(7): 672–79. doi: 10.1093/aje/kwi085.

p. 144: Cook, Marc D., Jacob M. Allen, Brandt D. Pence, Matthew A. Wallig, H. Rex Gaskins, Bryan A. White, and Jeffrey A. Woods. Exercise and gut immune function: Evidence of alterations in colon immune cell homeostasis and microbiome characteristics with exercise training. *Immunology and Cell Biology.* Dec 2015, doi:10.1038/icb.2015.108.

p. 145: "Sitting disease" by the numbers. http://www.juststand.org/tabid/674/language/en-us/default.aspx.

Vlahos, J. Is sitting a lethal activity? Apr 14, 2011. *New York Times.* http://www.nytimes.com/2011/04/magazine/mag-17sitting -t.html?pagewaned=print.

Watson, S. Too much sitting linked to an early death. *Harvard Health Publications.* http://www.health.harvard.edu/blog/too -much-sitting-linked-to-an-early death-201401297004.

p. 148: Adamson S., et al. High intensity training improves health and physical function in middle-aged adults. *Biology.* 2014, 3: 333–44, doi:10.3390/biology302333.

Hagerman, F. C., et al. Effects of high intensity resistance training on untrained older men: Strength, cardiovascular, and metabolic responses. *Journals of Gerontology.* Series A: Biological Sciences, Medical Sciences, 2000, 55(7): B336–46, doi:10.1093 /Gerona/55.7.B336.

p. 167: Creswell, J. David, Adrienne A. Taren, Emily K. Lindsay, Carol M. Greco, Peter J. Gianaros, April Fairgrieve, Anna L. Marsland, Kirk Warren Brown, Baldwin M. Way, Rhonda K. Rosen, and Jennifer L. Ferris. Alterations in resting-state functional connectivity link mindfulness meditation with reduced interleukin-6: A randomized controlled trial. *Biological Psychiatry.* Jul 1, 2016, 80(1): 53–61, doi:http://dx.doi .org/10.1016/j.biopsych.2016.01.008.

Kaliman, Perla, María Jesús Álvarez-López, Marta Cosín-Tomás, Melissa A. Rosenkranz, Antoine Lutz, and Richard J. Davidson. Rapid changes in histone deacetylases and inflammatory gene expression in expert meditators. *Psychoneuroendocrinology.* Feb 2014 (online: Nov 15, 2013), 40: 96–107, doi: 10.1016/j .psyneuen.2013.11.004.

Rath, Eva, and Dirk Haller. Mitochondria at the interface between danger signaling and metabolism: Role of unfolded protein responses in chronic inflammation. *Inflammatory Bowel Diseases.* Jul 2012, 18(7): 237.

Index

Note: Entries in *italics* indicate recipes.